RN Community Health Nursing
Review Module Edition 6.0

CONTRIBUTORS

Sheryl Sommer, PhD, RN, CNE
VP Nursing Education & Strategy

Janean Johnson, MSN, RN
Nursing Education Strategist

Karin Roberts, PhD, MSN, RN, CNE
Nursing Education Coordinator

Sharon R. Redding, EdD, RN, CNE
Nursing Education Specialist and Content Project Coordinator

Lois Churchill, MN, RN
Nursing Education Specialist

Carrie B. Elkins, DHSc, MSN, BC
Nursing Education Specialist

EDITORIAL AND PUBLISHING

Derek Prater
Spring Lenox
Michelle Renner
Mandy Tallmadge
Kelly Von Lunen

CONSULTANTS

Honey C. Holman, MSN, RN

Intellectual Property Notice

Important Notice to the Reader

User's Guide

Welcome to the Assessment Technologies Institute® RN Community Health Nursing Review Module Edition 6.0. The mission of ATI's Content Mastery Series® review modules is to provide user-friendly compendiums of nursing knowledge that will:

- Help you locate important information quickly.

- Assist in your learning efforts.

- Provide exercises for applying your nursing knowledge.

- Facilitate your entry into the nursing profession as a newly licensed RN.

Organization

Chapters in this review module use a nursing concepts organizing framework, beginning with an overview describing the central concept and its relevance to nursing. Subordinate themes are covered in outline form to demonstrate relationships and present the information in a clear, succinct manner. Some chapters have sections that group related concepts and contain their own overviews. These sections are included in the table of contents.

Application Exercises

Questions are provided at the end of each chapter so you can practice applying your knowledge. The Application Exercises include NCLEX-style questions, such as multiple-choice and multiple-select items, and questions that ask you to apply your knowledge in other formats, such as by using an ATI Active Learning Template. After the Application Exercises, an answer key is provided, along with rationales for the answers.

NCLEX® Connections

To prepare for the NCLEX-RN, it is important for you to understand how the content in this review module is connected to the NCLEX-RN test plan. You can find information on the detailed test plan at the National Council of State Boards of Nursing's Web site: https://www.ncsbn.org/. When reviewing content in this review module, regularly ask yourself, "How does this content fit into the test plan, and what types of questions related to this content should I expect?"

To help you in this process, we've included NCLEX Connections at the beginning of each unit and with each question in the Application Exercises Answer Keys. The NCLEX Connections at the beginning of each unit will point out areas of the detailed test plan that relate to the content within that unit. The NCLEX Connections attached to the Application Exercises Answer Keys will demonstrate how each exercise fits within the detailed content outline.

These NCLEX Connections will help you understand how the detailed content outline is organized, starting with major client needs categories and subcategories and followed by related content areas and tasks. The major client needs categories are:

- Safe and Effective Care Environment
  - Management of Care
  - Safety and Infection Control
- Health Promotion and Maintenance
- Psychosocial Integrity
- Physiological Integrity
  - Basic Care and Comfort
  - Pharmacological and Parenteral Therapies
  - Reduction of Risk Potential
  - Physiological Adaptation

An NCLEX Connection might, for example, alert you that content within a unit is related to:

- Safety and Infection Control
  - Home Safety
    - Assess need for client home modifications.

QSEN Competencies

As you use the review modules, you will note the integration of the Quality and Safety Education for Nurses (QSEN) competencies throughout the chapters. These competencies are integral components of the curriculum of many nursing programs in the United States and prepare you to provide safe, high-quality care as a newly licensed RN. Icons appear to draw your attention to the six QSEN competencies:

- Safety: The minimization of risk factors that could cause injury or harm while promoting quality care and maintaining a secure environment for clients, self, and others.

- Patient-Centered Care: The provision of caring and compassionate, culturally sensitive care that addresses clients' physiological, psychological, sociological, spiritual, and cultural needs, preferences, and values.

- Evidence-Based Practice: The use of current knowledge from research and other credible sources, on which to base clinical judgment and client care.

- Informatics: The use of information technology as a communication and information-gathering tool that supports clinical decision-making and scientifically based nursing practice.

- Quality Improvement: Care related and organizational processes that involve the development and implementation of a plan to improve health care services and better meet clients' needs.

- Teamwork and Collaboration: The delivery of client care in partnership with multidisciplinary members of the health care team to achieve continuity of care and positive client outcomes.

Icons

Icons are used throughout the review module to draw your attention to particular areas. Keep an eye out for these icons:

 This icon is used for NCLEX connections.

 This icon is used for content related to safety and is a QSEN competency. When you see this icon, take note of safety concerns or steps that nurses can take to ensure client safety and a safe environment.

 This icon is a QSEN competency that indicates the importance of a holistic approach to providing care.

 This icon, a QSEN competency, points out the integration of research into clinical practice.

 This icon is a QSEN competency and highlights the use of information technology to support nursing practice.

 This icon is used to focus on the QSEN competency of integrating planning processes to meet clients' needs.

 This icon highlights the QSEN competency of care delivery using an interprofessional approach.

This icon indicates that a media supplement, such as a graphic, animation, or video, is available. If you have an electronic copy of the review module, this icon will appear alongside clickable links to media supplements. If you have a hardcopy version of the review module, visit www.atitesting. com for details on how to access these features.

Feedback

ATI welcomes feedback regarding this review module. Please provide comments to: comments@atitesting.com.

TABLE OF CONTENTS

CHAPTER 1   Overview of Community Health Nursing

When reviewing the chapters in this unit, keep in mind the relevant sections of the NCLEX® outline, in particular:

Client Needs: Management of Care

› Relevant topics/tasks include:

» Advocacy

› Utilize advocacy resources appropriately.

» Ethical Practice

› Practice in a manner consistent with the code of ethics for registered nurses.

Client Needs: Health Promotion and Maintenance

› Relevant topics/tasks include:

» Health Promotion/Disease Prevention

› Assess and teach clients about health risks based on family, population, and/or community characteristics.

» Health Screening

› Perform targeted screening assessments (e.g., vision, hearing, nutrition).

chapter 1

Overview

- Community health nursing is a broad field that allows nurses to practice in a wide variety of settings.
- Community health nurses promote the health and welfare of clients across the lifespan and from diverse populations.
- Nurses working in the community should have an understanding of:
    - The foundations of community health nursing
    - The principles of community health nursing
    - Health promotion and disease prevention

FOUNDATIONS OF COMMUNITY HEALTH NURSING

Overview

- Various theories and specific definitions of care guide nursing practice in the community.

Community Health Nursing Theories

- Nursing theory provides the basis for care of the community and family. Theorists have developed sound principles to guide nurses in providing high-quality care. Examples of nursing theories appropriate for community health include the following:

THEORY/MODEL	DESCRIPTIONS
Nightingale's Theory of Environment	› Highlights the relationship between an individual's environment and health › Depicts health as a continuum › Emphasizes preventive care

Health Belief Model	› Purpose is to predict or explain health behaviors
	› Assumes that preventive health behaviors are taken primarily for the purpose of avoiding disease
	› Emphasizes change at the individual level
	› Describes the likelihood of taking an action to avoid disease based on:
	  » Perceived susceptibility, seriousness, and threat of a disease
	  » Modifying factors (e.g., demographics, knowledge level)
	  » Cues to action (e.g., media campaigns, disease impact on family/friends, recommendations from health care professionals)
	  » Perceived benefits minus perceived barriers to taking action

Milio's Framework for Prevention	› Complements the health belief model › Emphasizes change at the community level › Identifies relationship between health deficits and availability of health-promoting resources › Theorizes that behavior changes within a large number of people can ultimately lead to social change

Essentials of Community Nursing

- A community is a group of people and institutions that share geographic, civic, and/or social parameters.
- Communities vary in their characteristics and health needs.
- A community's health is determined by the degree to which the community's collective health needs are identified and met.
- Health indicators (mortality rates, disease prevalence, levels of physical activity, obesity, tobacco use, substance use) are often used to describe the health status of a community and serve as targets for the improvement of a community's health.
- Community health nurses are nurses who practice in the community. They usually have a facility from which they work (community health clinic, county health department), but their practice is not limited to institutional settings.

- The community or a population (an aggregate who shares one or more personal characteristics) within the community is the "client" in community health nursing.
- Community partnership occurs when community members, agencies, and businesses actively participate in the processes of health promotion and disease prevention. The development of community partnerships is critical to the accomplishment of health promotion and disease prevention strategies.
- Assessing to determine needs and intervening to protect and promote health, and preventing disease within a specific population (individuals at risk for hypertension, individuals without health insurance, individuals with a specific knowledge deficit) are the purposes of population-focused nursing.

COMMUNITY-BASED NURSING	
Focus of Care	› Individuals › Families
Nursing Activities	› Illness care: Management of acute and chronic conditions in settings where individuals, families, and groups live, work, and "attend" (schools, camps, prisons)
COMMUNITY-ORIENTED NURSING	
Focus of Care	› At-risk individuals, families, and groups › Community
Nursing Activities	› Health care: Determining health needs of a community, and intervening at the individual, family, and group level to improve the collective health of the community
COMMUNITY HEALTH NURSING PRACTICE	
Focus of Care	› Synthesis of nursing and public health theory
Nursing Activities	› Promote, preserve, and maintain the health of populations by the delivery of health services to individuals, families, and groups in order to impact "community health."
PUBLIC HEALTH NURSING PRACTICE	
Focus of Care	› Synthesis of nursing and public health theory
Nursing Activities	› Promote, preserve, and maintain the health of populations through disease and disability prevention and health protection of the community as a whole. › Core functions » Systematic assessment of the health of populations » Development of policies to support the health of populations » Ensuring that essential health services are available to all persons

---

PRINCIPLES OF COMMUNITY HEALTH NURSING

Overview

- Principles guiding community health nursing practice include the following:
  - Ethical Considerations
  - Advocacy
  - Epidemiology
  - Epidemiological Calculations
  - Epidemiological Triangle
  - The Epidemiological Process
  - Community-Based Health Education

Ethical Considerations

- The Public Health Code of Ethics identifies the ethical practice of public health. Ethical considerations include preventing harm, doing no harm, promoting good, respecting both individual and community rights, respecting autonomy and diversity, and providing confidentiality, competency, trustworthiness, and advocacy.

- Community health nurses are concerned with protecting, promoting, preserving, and maintaining health, as well as preventing disease. These concerns reflect the ethical principle of promoting good and preventing harm. Balancing individual rights versus rights of community groups is a challenge.

- Community health nurses address the challenges of autonomy and providing ethical care. Client rights include the right to information disclosure, privacy, informed consent, information confidentiality, and participation in treatment decisions.

APPLICATION OF ETHICAL PRINCIPLES TO COMMUNITY HEALTH NURSING		
	DEFINITION	**SITUATIONS**
Respect for Autonomy	› Individuals select those actions that fulfill their goals.	› Respecting a client's right to self-determination (making a decision not to pursue chemotherapy)
Nonmaleficence	› No harm is done when applying standards of care.	› Developing plans of care that include a system for monitoring and evaluating outcomes
Beneficence	› Maximize possible benefits and minimize possible harms.	› Assessing risks and benefits when planning interventions
Distributive Justice	› Fair distribution of the benefits and burden in society is based on the needs and contributions of its members.	› Determining eligibility for health care services based on income and fiscal resources

Advocacy

- Client advocate is one role of the community health nurse. The nurse plays the role of informer, supporter, and mediator for the client. The following are basic to client advocacy.

  - Clients are autonomous beings who have the right to make decisions affecting their own health and welfare.

  - Clients have the right to expect a nurse-client relationship that is based on trust, collaboration, and shared respect, related to health, and considerate of their thoughts and feelings.

  - Clients are responsible for their own health.

  - It is the nurse's responsibility to advocate for resources or services that meet the client's health care needs.

  - Advocating for clients requires assertiveness, placing priority on the client's values, and willingness to progress through the chain of command for resolution.

Epidemiology

- Epidemiology is the study of health-related trends in populations for the purposes of disease prevention, health maintenance, and health protection.

- Epidemiology relies on statistical evidence to determine the rate of spread of disease and the proportion of people affected. It also is used to evaluate the effectiveness of disease prevention and health promotion activities and to determine the extent to which goals have been met.

- Epidemiology provides a broad understanding of the spread, transmission, and incidence of disease and injury. This information is an important component of community assessment and program planning.

- Community health nurses are in the unique position of being able to identify cases, recognize patterns of disease, eliminate barriers to disease control, and provide education and counseling targeted at a disease condition or specific risk factors.

- Epidemiology involves the study of the relationships among an agent, a host, and an environment (referred to as the epidemiological triangle). Their interaction determines the development and cessation of communicable diseases, and they form a web of causality, which increases or decreases the risk for disease.

  - The agent is the animate or inanimate object that causes the disease.

  - The host is the living being that is affected by the agent.

  - The environment is the setting or surrounding that sustains the host.

Epidemiological Calculations

INCIDENCE
Number of new cases in the population at a specific time ÷ population total x 1,000 = _____ per 1,000

PREVALENCE
Number of existing cases in the population at a specific time ÷ population total x 1,000 = _____ per 1,000

CRUDE MORTALITY RATE
Number of deaths ÷ population total x 1,000 = _____ per 1,000

INFANT MORTALITY RATE
Number of infant deaths before 1 year of age in a year ÷ numbers of live births in the same year x 1,000 = _____ per 1,000

ATTACK RATE
Number of people exposed to a specific agent who develop the disease ÷ total number of people exposed

- An epidemic is when the rate of disease exceeds the usual level of the condition in a defined population.

The Epidemiological Process

PHASE	DESCRIPTION
Determine the nature, extent, and possible significance of the problem.	› During this phase of the process, the nurse collects information from as many sources as possible. This information is then used to determine the scope of the problem.
Using the gathered data, formulate a possible theory.	› At this time, the nurse projects and explores the possible explanations.
Gather information from a variety of sources in order to narrow down the possibilities.	› The nurse assesses all possible sites for amassing information related to the disease process. The nurse evaluates the plausibility of the proposed hypothesis.
Make the plan.	› In this phase of the process, the nurse focuses on breaking the cycle of disease. All factors influencing the spread of the disease must be considered and identified. Priorities are established to break the chain of transmission and to control the spread of the disease.
Put the plan into action.	› Using all available means, the nurse puts the plan for controlling the disease into action.
Evaluate the plan.	› The nurse gathers pertinent information to determine the success of the plan. Using this plan, the nurse evaluates the success in prevention of the spread of the disease.
Report and follow up.	› The nurse synthesizes evaluation data into a format that is understandable. Then nurse evaluates successes and failures and bases follow-up on the evaluation information.

EPIDEMIOLOGICAL TRIANGLE

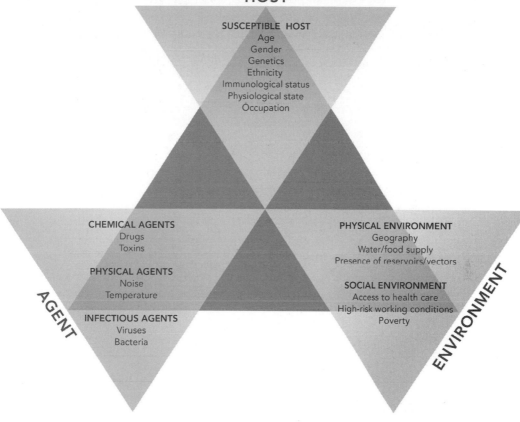

- Epidemiology involves the study of the relationships among an agent, a host, and an environment (referred to as the epidemiological triangle). Their interaction determines the development and cessation of communicable diseases, and they form a web of causality, which increases or decreases the risk for disease.

  ○ The agent is the animate or inanimate object that causes the disease.

  ○ The host is the living being that is affected by the agent.

  ○ The environment is the setting or surrounding that sustains the host.

Community Health Education

- Community health nurses regularly provide health education in order to promote, maintain, and restore the health of populations. This is accomplished through a variety of means, such as community education programs.

- In designing community education programs, nurses must take into account the barriers that make learning difficult. Some of these obstacles include age, cultural barriers, poor reading and comprehension skills, language barriers, barriers to access, and lack of motivation. Effective community health education requires planning.

- Learning Theories Used in Community Health Nursing

  ○ Behavioral theory – Use of reinforcement methods to change learners' behaviors.

  ○ Cognitive theory – Use of sensory input and repetition to change learners' patterns of thought, thereby changing behaviors.

  ○ Critical theory – Use of ongoing discussion and inquiry to increase learners' depth of knowledge, thereby changing thinking and behaviors.

  ○ Developmental theory – Use of techniques specific to learners' developmental stages to determine readiness to learn, and to impart knowledge.

  ○ Humanistic theory – Assists learners to grow by emphasizing emotions and relationships and believing that free choice will prompt actions that are in their own best interest.

  ○ Social learning theory – Links information to beliefs and values to change or shift the learners' expectations.

- Learning Styles

  ○ Community health nurses enhance the provision of education by addressing learning styles.

    ▪ Visual learners learn through "seeing" and methods such as note taking, video viewing, and presentations. These learners "think in pictures."

    ▪ Auditory learners learn through "listening" and methods such as verbal lectures, discussion, and reading aloud. These learners "interpret meaning while listening."

    ▪ Tactile-kinesthetic learners learn through "doing" and methods such as trial and error, hands-on approaches, and return demonstration. These learners gain "meaning through exploration."

- Development of a Community Health Education Plan

  ○ First, identify population-specific learning needs.

  ○ Consider population-specific concerns and effect of health needs on the population to determine the priority learning need.

  ○ Select aspects of learning theories (behavioral, cognitive, critical, developmental, humanistic, social learning) to use in the educational program based on the identified learning need.

  ○ Identify barriers to learning, and learning styles (visual, auditory, tactile-kinesthetic).

  ○ Design the educational program.

    ▪ Set short- and long-term learning objectives that are measurable and achievable.

    ▪ Select an appropriate educational method based on learning objectives and assessment of participants' learning styles.

- Select content appropriate to learning objectives and allotted time frame.
- Select an evaluation method that will provide feedback regarding achievement of short-term learning objectives, and long-term impact on behavior.

○ Implement the education program. Ensure an environment that is conducive to learning (minimal distractions, favorable to interaction, learner comfort, readability).

○ Evaluate the achievement of learning objectives and the effectiveness of instruction.

HEALTH PROMOTION AND DISEASE PREVENTION

Overview

- National health goals guide nurses in developing health promotion strategies to improve individual and community health.
- Community health nurses participate in three levels of prevention – primary, secondary, and tertiary.

Health Promotion

- National health goals are derived from scientific data and trends collected during the prior decade. These goals are based on those issues that are considered major risks to the health and wellness of the United States' population.

  ○ *Healthy People* was initiated in 1979, and every 10 years, publishes the national health objectives that serve as a guide for promoting health and preventing disease.

  ○ *Healthy People* is coordinated by the United States Department of Health and Human Services, along with other federal agencies, and transitioned to *Healthy People 2020* in January 2010.

- National health goals guide the nurse in developing health promotion strategies to improve individual and community health.
- The community health nurse actively helps people to change their lifestyles in order to move toward a state of optimal health (physical and psychosocial).
- Preventive services include health education and counseling, immunizations, and other actions that aim to prevent a potential disease or disability.
- The community health nurse provides preventive services in multiple community settings.
- The community health nurse is often responsible for planning and implementing screening programs for at-risk populations.
- Successful screening programs provide accurate, reliable results, can be inexpensively and quickly administered to large groups, and produce few if any side effects.

 View Video: Levels of Prevention

Disease Prevention

LEVELS OF PREVENTION		
FOCUS	**EXAMPLES OF COMMUNITY HEALTH NURSE PREVENTION ACTIVITIES**	
Primary Prevention		
› Prevention of the initial occurrence of disease or injury	› Nutrition education › Family planning and sex education › Smoking cessation education › Communicable disease education › Education about health and hygiene issues to specific groups (day care workers, restaurant workers)	› Safety education (seat belt use, helmet use) › Prenatal classes › Providing immunizations › Advocating for access to health care, healthy environments
Secondary Prevention		

› Early detection and treatment of disease with the goal of limiting severity and adverse effects	› Community assessments
	› Disease surveillance (communicable diseases)
	› Screenings
	  » Cancer (breast, cervical, testicular, prostate, colorectal)
	  » Diabetes mellitus
	  » Hypertension
		» Hypercholesterolemia
		» Sensory impairments
		» Tuberculosis
		» Lead exposure
		» Genetic disorders/metabolic deficiencies in newborns
		› Control of outbreaks of communicable diseases

Tertiary Prevention		
› Maximization of recovery after an injury or illness (rehabilitation)	› Nutrition counseling › Exercise rehabilitation › Case management (chronic illness, mental illness)	› Physical and occupational therapy › Support groups › Exercise for hypertensive clients (individual)

APPLICATION EXERCISES

1. A nurse manager at a community agency is developing an orientation program for newly hired nurses. When discussing the differences between community-based and community-oriented nursing, the nurse should include which of the following as examples of community-based nursing? (Select all that apply.)

_____ A. A home health nurse performing wound care for a client who is immobile

_____ B. An occupational health nurse providing classes on body mechanics at a local industrial plant

C. A school nurse teaching a student who has asthma about medications

_____ D. A parish nurse teaching a class on low-sodium cooking techniques

_____ E. A mental health nurse discussing stress management techniques with a support group

2. A nurse is advocating for local leaders to place a newly approved community health clinic in an area of the city that has fewer resources than other areas. The nurse is advocating for the leaders to uphold which of the following ethical principles?

A. Distributive justice

B. Fidelity

C. Respect for autonomy

D. Veracity

3. A nurse is preparing an education program on disease transmission for employees at a local day care facility. When discussing the epidemiological triangle, the nurse should include which of the following as agents? (Select all that apply.)

_____ A. Resource availability

_____ B. Ethnicity

_____ C. Toxins

_____ D. Bacteria

_____ E. Altered immunity

4. A nurse is developing a community health education program for a group of clients who have a new diagnosis of diabetes mellitus. Which of the following learning strategies should the nurse include for clients who are auditory learners?

    A. Showing informational videos

    B. Providing equipment to practice hands-on skills

    C. Supplying outlines for note-taking

    D. Facilitating small group discussions

5. A community health nurse is implementing health programs with several populations in the local area. In which of the following situations is the nurse using primary prevention?

    A. Performing a home safety check at a client's home

    B. Teaching healthy nutrition to clients who have hypertension

    C. Providing influenza immunizations to employees at a local preschool

    D. Implementing a program to notify individuals exposed to a communicable disease

6. A school nurse is planning prevention activities for students within the school system. Using the ATI Active Learning Template: Basic Concept complete this item to include the following:

    A. Related Content:
- Define primary prevention
- Define secondary prevention
- Define tertiary prevention

    B. Nursing Interventions:
- Two primary prevention activities the nurse should plan
- Two secondary prevention activities the nurse should plan
- Two tertiary prevention activities the nurse should plan

APPLICATION EXERCISES KEY

1.   A. **CORRECT:** This is an example of community-based nursing, which involves management of acute and chronic conditions in a community setting.

   B. INCORRECT: This is an example of community-oriented nursing, which involves health care of individuals, families and groups to improve the collective health of the community.

   C. **CORRECT:** This is an example of community-based nursing, which involves management of acute and chronic conditions in a community setting.

   D. INCORRECT: This is an example of community-oriented nursing, which involves health care of individuals, families and groups to improve the collective health of the community.

   E. INCORRECT: This is an example of community-oriented nursing, which involves health care of individuals, families and groups to improve the collective health of the community.

   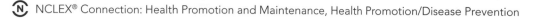 NCLEX® Connection: Health Promotion and Maintenance, Health Promotion/Disease Prevention

2.   A. **CORRECT:** The nurse is advocating for the leaders to uphold the ethical principle of distributive justice, which is the fair distribution of benefits and burden in society.

   B. INCORRECT: The nurse is not advocating for the leaders to uphold the ethical principle of fidelity, which involves keeping commitments and following through with promises.

   C. INCORRECT: The nurse is not advocating for the leaders to uphold the ethical principle of respect for autonomy, which is supporting the rights of individuals to determine and pursue personal health care goals.

   D. INCORRECT: The nurse is not advocating for the leaders to uphold the ethical principle of veracity, which is the concept of telling the truth.

   NCLEX® Connection: Management of Care, Ethical Practice

3.   A. INCORRECT: The nurse should include resource availability as an environmental factor when discussing the epidemiological triangle.

    B. INCORRECT: The nurse should include ethnicity as a host factor when discussing the epidemiological triangle.

    C. **CORRECT:** The nurse should include toxins as an agent when discussing the epidemiological triangle.

    D. **CORRECT:** The nurse should include bacteria as an agent when discussing the epidemiological triangle.

    E. INCORRECT: The nurse should include altered immunity as a host factor when discussing the epidemiological triangle.

 NCLEX® Connection: Safety and Infection Control, Standard Precautions/Transmission-Based Precautions/Surgical Asepsis

4.   A. INCORRECT: Showing informational videos is an appropriate learning strategy for clients who are visual learners.

    B. INCORRECT: Providing equipment to practice hands-on skills is an appropriate learning strategy for clients who are tactile-kinesthetic learners.

    C. INCORRECT: Supplying outlines for note-taking is an appropriate learning strategy for clients who are visual learners.

    D. **CORRECT:** Facilitating small group discussions is an appropriate learning strategy for clients who are auditory learners.

 NCLEX® Connection: Health Promotion and Maintenance, Health Promotion/Disease Prevention

5.   A. INCORRECT: The nurse is using secondary prevention when performing a home safety check at a client's home.

    B. INCORRECT: The nurse is using tertiary prevention when teaching healthy nutrition to clients who have hypertension.

    C. **CORRECT:** The nurse is using primary prevention when providing influenza immunizations to employees at a local preschool.

    D. INCORRECT: The nurse is using secondary prevention when implementing a program to notify individuals exposed to a communicable disease.

 NCLEX® Connection: Health Promotion and Maintenance, Health Promotion/Disease Prevention

6. *Using the ATI Active Learning Template: Basic Concept*

A. Related Content

- Primary Prevention – Strategies that prevent the initial occurrence of disease or injury
- Secondary Prevention – Strategies that lead to early detection and treatment of disease with the goal of limiting severity and adverse effects
- Tertiary Prevention – Strategies that maximize recovery after an injury or illness

B. Nursing Interventions

- Primary Prevention Activities
  - Teaching healthy heart curriculum (nutrition, exercise, not smoking)
  - Educating about dental health
  - Discussing safety (seat belts, bicycle helmets, stranger safety)
  - Administering immunizations
  - Teaching about communicable disease transmission
  - Sex education
  - Advocating for safe playground equipment
  - Substance use prevention education
- Secondary Prevention Activities
  - Performing tuberculin skin tests
  - Performing routine checks for pediculosis
  - Taking measures to control communicable disease outbreaks
  - Screening for lead exposure
  - Implementing scoliosis screenings
  - Identifying students at risk for suicide or self-harm
  - Performing vision and hearing screenings
  - Checking heights and weights
  - Identifying child abuse or neglect
- Tertiary Prevention Activities
  - Teaching about allergic triggers for students with asthma
  - Administering medications to treat chronic conditions (asthma, diabetes, seizure disorders)
  - Monitoring glucose levels and administering insulin to students who have diabetes
  - Discussing and planning for nutritional needs of students who have diabetes
  - Developing communication methods for students with autism

Ⓝ NCLEX® Connection: Health Promotion and Maintenance, Health Promotion/Disease Prevention

NCLEX® CONNECTIONS

When reviewing the chapters in this unit, keep in mind the relevant sections of the NCLEX® outline, in particular:

Client Needs: Management of Care

› Relevant topics/tasks include:
  » Continuity of Care
    › Maintain continuity of care between/among health care agencies.

Client Needs: Health Promotion and Maintenance

› Relevant topics/tasks include:
  » Aging Process
    › Assess client reactions to expected age-related changes.
  » Developmental Stages and Transitions
    › Recognize cultural and religious influences that may impact family functioning.
  » Health Promotion/Disease Prevention
    › Identify risk factors for disease/illness.

Client Needs: Psychosocial Integrity

› Relevant topics/tasks include:
  » Cultural Diversity
    › Respect the cultural background/practices of the client.

Overview

- Family and culture, social and environmental factors, access to health care, and health care financing all influence community health.

- Culture is the beliefs, values, attitudes, and behaviors shared by a group of people and transmitted from generation to generation.

- Environmental health refers to the influence of environmental conditions on the development of disease or injury.

- Access to health care is impacted by the availability of services in a community, as well as individual, family, and community circumstances.

Family and Cultural Care

- Congruency between culture and health care is essential to the well-being of the client. The link between health beliefs and practices is greatly influenced by an individual's culture.

Q
PCC

- It is important to assess cultural beliefs and practices when developing a plan of care.

  ○ Community health nurses need to consider that there are variations within each culture.

  ○ The uniqueness of each client needs to be considered.

  ○ Community health nurses should be familiar with cultures represented in the local community.

- Acculturation is the process of merging with or adopting the traits of a different culture. Adapting to a new culture requires changes in daily living practices. These changes relate to language, education, work, recreation, social experiences, and the health care system.

- Cultural awareness includes self-awareness of one's own cultural background, biases, and differences. Culturally aware nurses are:

  ○ More likely to explore cultural variations among clients.

  ○ Better able to understand how personal beliefs impact client care.

  ○ Able to recognize the meaning of health differs with each culture.

- Cultural needs of the client are as important as physical and psychological needs. Personal cultural values should not be imposed on the client, and nurses should avoid ethnocentrism and stereotyping in the provision of care.

- Cultural competence involves respecting personal dignity and preferences, as well as acknowledging cultural differences. The provision of culturally competent care requires nurses to be responsive to the needs of clients from different cultures.

Cultural Assessment

- A cultural assessment provides information to the health care provider about the effect of culture on communication, space and physical contact, time, social organization, and environmental control factors.
  - General cultural-assessment parameters
    - Ethnic background
    - Religious preferences
    - Family structure
    - Language
    - Communication needs
    - Education
    - Cultural values
    - Food patterns
    - Health practices
  - The three steps of data collection
    - Collection of self-identifying data about the client's ethnic background, religious preference, family structure, food patterns, and health practices.
    - Posing questions that address the client's perceptions of his health needs.
    - Identification of how cultural factors may impact the effectiveness of nursing interventions.

Using an Interpreter

- An interpreter should be used when it is difficult for a nurse or client to understand the other's language.
- Interpreters should have knowledge of health-related terminology.
- The use of family members as interpreters is not advisable because clients may need privacy in discussing sensitive matters.
- Client preferences should be considered when selecting the age and sex of interpreters.
- Interpreters should not be from the same community as the client.
- Health teaching materials should be available in the client's primary language.
- Federal government mandates require agencies to have a plan that will improve access to federal health care programs for individuals with limited English proficiency.

Cultural Competence: Areas for Self-Assessment

- Am I aware of my culture and views about other cultures?
- Am I able to perform a culturally sensitive assessment?
- Do I have the knowledge necessary to develop culturally appropriate nursing interventions?
- What is my goal in learning about diverse populations?

Conveying Cultural Sensitivity

- The nurse should:
  - Address clients by their last names, unless the client gives the nurse permission to use other names.
  - Introduce himself by name and explain his position.
  - Be authentic and honest about what he does or does not know about a client's culture.
  - Use language that is culturally sensitive.
  - Find out what clients know about their health problems and treatments, and assess cultural congruence.
  - Incorporate clients' preferences and practices into care when possible.
  - Not make assumptions about clients.
  - Encourage clients to ask about anything that they may not understand.
  - Respect clients' values, beliefs, and practices.
  - Show respect for clients' support systems.

Environmental Risks

- Toxins, such as lead, pesticides, mercury, solvents, asbestos, and radon.
- Air pollution, such as carbon monoxide, particulate matter, ozone, lead, aerosols, nitrogen dioxide, sulfur dioxide, and tobacco smoke.
- Water pollution, such as wastes, erosion after mining or timbering, and run-off from chemicals added to the soil.

Roles for Nurses in Environmental Health

- Facilitate public participation.
- Perform individual and population risk assessments.
- Implement risk communication.
- Conduct epidemiological investigations.
- Participate in policy development.

Assessment of Environmental Health

- The "I PREPARE" mnemonic is one method of determining current and past environmental exposures.
  - I = Investigate potential exposures
  - P = Present work (exposures, use of personal protective equipment, location of material safety data sheets [MSDS], taking home exposures, trends)
  - R = Residence (age of home, heating, recent remodeling, chemical storage, water)
  - E = Environmental concerns (air, water, soil, industries in neighborhood, waste site or landfill nearby)
  - P = Past work (exposures, farm work, military, volunteer, seasonal, length of work)

- ○ A = Activities (hobbies, activities, gardening, fishing, hunting, soldering, melting, burning, eating, pesticides, alternative healing/medicines)

- ○ R = Referrals and resources (Environmental Protection Agency, Agency for Toxic Substances & Disease Registry, Association of Occupational and Environmental Clinics, MSDS, OSHA, local health department, environmental agency, poison control)

- ○ E = Educate (risk reduction, prevention, follow-up)

- Key Questions for Environmental Health History

  - ○ Housing: What is the physical condition of residence, age, location, school, day care, or work site? Are lighting, ventilation, and heating/cooling systems adequate?

  - ○ What are the occupations of household members (current and past, longest-held jobs)?

  - ○ Is tobacco smoke present?

  - ○ Are there any recent home remodeling activities, such as the installation of new carpet or furniture or refinishing of furniture?

  - ○ What hobbies are done in the home?

  - ○ Is there any other recent exposure to chemicals or radiation?

  - ○ Are pets present in the home, and are they healthy?

  - ○ Has there been any lead exposure in old paint, crafts, leaded pottery, or dishes?

  - ○ What is the source and quality of the drinking water?

  - ○ How is sewage and waste disposed of in the home?

  - ○ Are there pesticides used around the home or garden? Is there any evidence of mold or fungi?

  - ○ Where do children play? Is there any hazardous play equipment or toys?

  - ○ Does the surrounding neighborhood present any hazards with closeness to highways or small businesses, such as dry cleaning, photo processing, industry, or auto repair?

National Health Care Goals

- Reductions in:
  - ○ Toxic air emissions
  - ○ Waterborne disease outbreaks
  - ○ Per capita domestic water use
  - ○ Blood lead levels in children
  - ○ Pesticide exposures requiring visits to health care facility
  - ○ Indoor allergen levels
  - ○ U.S. homes with lead-based paint or related hazards
  - ○ Exposure to chemicals and pollutants
  - ○ Risks posed by hazardous sites
  - ○ Number of new schools near highways
  - ○ Global burden of disease due to environmental concerns

- Increases in:
  - Use of alternative modes of transportation for work
  - Number of days that beaches are open and safe for swimming
  - Recycling of municipal solid waste
  - Testing for presence of lead-based paint in pre-1978 housing
  - Monitoring for diseases or conditions caused by environmental hazards
  - Homes with radon mitigation (those at-risk) & radon-reducing features
  - Schools with policies/practices to promote health/safety
  - Presence/use of information systems related to environmental health

Environmental Health Nursing Interventions

PRIMARY PREVENTION	
Individual	› Educate individuals to reduce environmental hazards.
Community	› Educate groups to reduce environmental hazards. › Advocate for safe air and water. › Support programs for waste reduction and recycling. › Advocate for waste reduction and effective waste management.
SECONDARY PREVENTION	
Individual	› Survey for health conditions that may be related to environmental and occupational exposures. › Obtain environmental health histories of individuals. › Monitor workers for levels of chemical exposures at job sites. › Screen children 6 months to 5 years old for blood lead levels.
Community	› Survey for health conditions that may be related to environmental and occupational exposures. › Assess homes, schools, work sites, and the community for environmental hazards.
TERTIARY PREVENTION	
Individual	› Refer homeowners to lead abatement resources. › Educate asthmatic clients about environmental triggers.
Community	› Become active in consumer and health-related organizations and legislation related to environmental health issues. › Support cleanup of toxic waste sites and removal of other hazards.

Access to Health Care

- Community health nurses must advocate for improved access to health care services.

- Community assessment includes evaluating the adequacy of health services within the community and the accessibility of those services by those needing access.

- It is important to identify barriers that community members, particularly vulnerable populations, encounter when accessing health services.

- Barriers to health care include:

  ○ Inadequate health care insurance

  ○ Inability to pay for health care services

  ○ Language barriers

  ○ Cultural barriers

  ○ Lack of health care providers in a community

  ○ Geographic isolation

  ○ Social isolation

  ○ Lack of communication tools (e.g., telephones)

  ○ Lack of personal or public transportation to health care facilities

  ○ Inconvenient hours

  ○ Attitudes of health care personnel toward clients of low socioeconomic status or those with different cultural/ethnic backgrounds

  ○ Eligibility requirements for state/federal assistance programs

Health Care Organizations and Financing

- International Health Organizations

  ○ World Health Organization (WHO)

    ▪ Provides daily information regarding the occurrence of internationally important diseases.

    ▪ Establishes world standards for antibiotics and vaccines.

    ▪ The WHO primarily focuses on the health care workforce and education, environment, sanitation, infectious diseases, maternal and child health, and primary care.

- Federal Health Agencies

  ○ U.S. Department of Health & Human Services

    ▪ Under the direction of the Secretary of Health

    ▪ Funded through federal taxes

- Consists of the following agencies:
  - Administration for Children and Families (ACF)
  - Administration for Community Living (ACL)
  - Centers for Medicare and Medicaid Services (CMS) – Also administers the Health Insurance Portability and Accountability Act (HIPAA), disability insurance, Aid to Families with Dependent Children (AFDC), and Supplemental Security Income (SSI).

MEDICARE	MEDICAID
› Individuals must be older than 65 years and receiving Social Security, have been receiving disability benefits for 2 years, have amyotrophic lateral sclerosis and receive disability benefits, or have kidney failure and be on maintenance dialysis or had a kidney transplant to qualify for Medicare.	› Medicaid provides health care coverage for individuals of low socioeconomic status and children, through the combined efforts of federal and state governments. Eligibility is based on household size and income, with priority given to children, pregnant women, and those who have a disability.
› Medicare includes four parts.	› Medicaid provides inpatient and outpatient hospital care, laboratory and radiology services, home health care, vaccines for children, family planning, pregnancy-related care, and Early and Periodic Screening, Diagnosis, and Treatment (EPSDT) services for those younger than 21 years.
» Part A (hospital care, home care, limited skilled nursing care)	
» Part B (medical care, diagnostic services, physiotherapy)	
» Part C (also known as the Medicare Advantage plan – is a combination of Part A and Part B and is provided through a private insurance company)	
» Part D (prescription drug coverage)	

  - Agency for Healthcare Research and Quality (AHRQ)
  - Centers for Disease Control and Prevention (CDC) – Works to prevent and control disease, injury, and disability both nationally and internationally.
  - Agency for Toxic Substances and Disease Registry (ATSDR)
  - Food and Drug Administration (FDA)
  - Health Resources and Service Administration (HRSA) – Includes the Division of Nursing, Division of Medicine and Dentistry, and the Division of Public Health and Interdisciplinary Education.
  - Indian Health Service (IHS)
  - National Institutes of Health (NIH) – Supports biomedical research and includes the National Institute of Nursing Research.
  - Substance Abuse and Mental Health Services Administration (SAMHSA)
- Veterans Health Administration (within the U.S. Department of Veterans Affairs) – Finances health services for active and retired military persons and dependents.

- ○ State Health Agencies
  - ▪ State Departments of Health
    - ▫ Manages the Women, Infants and Children (WIC) program.
    - ▫ Oversees Children's Health Insurance Program (CHIP), which offers expanded health coverage to uninsured children whose families do not qualify for Medicaid.
    - ▫ Establishes public health policies.
    - ▫ Provides assistance/support for local health departments.
    - ▫ Responsible for the administration of the Medicaid program.
    - ▫ Reports notifiable communicable disease within the state to the CDC.
  - ▪ State Boards of Nursing
    - ▫ Development and oversight of the state's nurse practice act.
    - ▫ Licensure of registered and licensed practical nurses.
    - ▫ Oversight of the state's schools of nursing.
- Local Health Department
  - ○ The primary focus of a local health department is the health of its citizens.
  - ○ Local health departments offer various services and programs.
  - ○ Responsible for identifying and intervening to meet health needs of the local community.
  - ○ Work closely with local officials, businesses, and stakeholders.
  - ○ Report notifiable communicable diseases to state departments of health.
  - ○ Nurses at the community level typically function in the nursing roles of caregiver, advocate, teacher, coordinator, and consultant.
  - ○ Funded through local taxes with support from federal and state funds.
- Private Funding
  - ○ Health insurance
  - ○ Employer benefits
  - ○ Managed care
    - ▪ Health maintenance organizations (HMOs) – Comprehensive care is provided to members by a set of designated providers.
    - ▪ Preferred provider organizations (PPOs) – Predetermined rates are set for services delivered to members; financial incentives are in place to promote use of PPO providers.
    - ▪ Medical savings accounts – Untaxed money is put in an account for use for medical expenses.

APPLICATION EXERCISES

1. A nurse is preparing an educational program on cultural perspectives in nursing. The nurse should include that which of the following are influenced by an individual's culture? (Select all that apply.)

_____ A. Nutritional practices

_____ B. Family structure

_____ C. Health care interactions

_____ D. Biological variations

_____ E. Views about illness

2. A nurse is caring for a client who is from a different culture than himself. When beginning the cultural assessment, which of the following actions should the nurse take first?

A. Determine the client's perception of his current health status.

B. Gather data about the client's cultural beliefs.

C. Determine how the client's culture may impact the effectiveness of nursing actions.

D. Gather information about previous client interactions with the health care system.

3. A nurse is using the I PREPARE mnemonic to assess a client's potential environmental exposures. Which of the following is an appropriate question for the nurse to ask to assess for "A" in the mnemonic?

A. "What do you like to do for fun?"

B. "What year was your residence built?"

C. "What jobs have you had in the past?"

D. "What industries are near where you live?"

4. A nurse is conducting health screenings at a statewide health fair and identifies several clients who require referral to a provider. Which of the following statements by a client indicates a barrier to accessing health care?

A. "I don't drive, and my son is only available to take me places in the mornings."

B. "I can't take off during the day and the local after-hours clinic is no longer in operation."

C. "Only one doctor in my town is a designated provider by my health maintenance organization."

D. "I would like to schedule an appointment with the local doctor in my town who speaks Spanish and English."

5. A nurse is interviewing for a position at the local health department. When preparing for the interview, the nurse should find that which of the following are responsibilities of this agency? (Select all that apply.)

_____ A. Managing the Women, Infants, and Children program

_____ B. Providing education to achieve community health goals

_____ C. Coordinating directives from state personnel

_____ D. Reporting communicable diseases to the CDC

_____ E. Licensing of registered nurses

6. A nurse is conducting an environmental health history during a postpartum home visit. Residents in the home include the mother, her partner, a 1-week-old infant, 2 year-old toddler, and 7-year-old child. Using the ATI Active Learning Template: Basic Concept and the ATI Community Health and Nursing Care of Children Review Modules, complete this item to include the following:

A. Underlying principles:

- Two national health goals that relate to this family

- Two questions to ask as part of the environmental health history

B. Nursing interventions: Two environmental health teaching points for this family

APPLICATION EXERCISES KEY

1. A. **CORRECT:** Culture is the beliefs, values, attitudes, and behaviors shared by a group of people and transmitted from generation to generation. Nutritional practices are influenced by an individual's culture.

    B. **CORRECT:** Culture is the beliefs, values, attitudes, and behaviors shared by a group of people and transmitted from generation to generation. Family structure is influenced by an individual's culture.

    C. **CORRECT:** Culture is the beliefs, values, attitudes, and behaviors shared by a group of people and transmitted from generation to generation. Health care interactions are influenced by an individual's culture.

    D. INCORRECT: Biological variations are physical, biological and physiological differences between races, and are not influenced by the beliefs, values, and attitudes of an individual.

    E. **CORRECT:** Culture is the beliefs, values, attitudes, and behaviors shared by a group of people and transmitted from generation to generation. Views about illness are influenced by an individual's culture.

    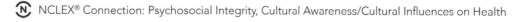 NCLEX® Connection: Psychosocial Integrity, Cultural Awareness/Cultural Influences on Health

2. A. INCORRECT: It is important for the nurse to determine the client's perception of his current health status. However, when conducting a cultural assessment, the nurse should perform a different action first.

    B. **CORRECT:** The nurse's first action when beginning a cultural assessment is to collect self-identifying data about the client, including specific information about how the client's cultural beliefs influence family structure, food patterns, religious preferences, and health practices.

    C. INCORRECT: While it is important for the nurse to determine how the client's culture may impact the effectiveness of nursing actions, the nurse must gather other information first.

    D. INCORRECT: It is important for the nurse to gather information about previous client interactions with the health care system. However, when conducting a cultural assessment, the nurse should perform a different action first.

    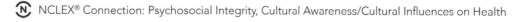 NCLEX® Connection: Psychosocial Integrity, Cultural Awareness/Cultural Influences on Health

3.   A. **CORRECT:** This is an appropriate question for the nurse to ask when assessing for "A," which represents activities in the mnemonic.

   B. INCORRECT: This is not an appropriate question for the nurse to ask when assessing for "A" in the mnemonic. This question is appropriate to assess the first "R," which represents residence in the mnemonic.

   C. INCORRECT: This is not an appropriate question for the nurse to ask when assessing for "A" in the mnemonic. This question is appropriate to assess the second "P," which represents past work in the mnemonic.

   D. INCORRECT: This is not an appropriate question for the nurse to ask when assessing for "A" in the mnemonic. This question is appropriate to assess the first "E," which represents environmental concerns in the mnemonic.

    NCLEX® Connection: Safety and Infection Control, Home Safety

4.   A. INCORRECT: The availability of a family member to provide transportation for a client in the morning is not a barrier to accessing health care. The follow-up appointment should be scheduled during this time frame.

   B. **CORRECT:** Inconvenient hours make scheduling a follow-up appointment challenging, and indicates a barrier to accessing health care for this client.

   C. INCORRECT: A single provider in the local community that is approved by the client's health maintenance organization does not indicate a barrier to accessing health care. The follow-up appointment should be scheduled with this provider.

   D. INCORRECT: A provider who is bilingual does not indicate a barrier to accessing health care. This increases accessibility for clients who may speak a different language.

    NCLEX® Connection: Health Promotion and Maintenance, Health Screening

5.   A. INCORRECT: Managing the Women, Infants, and Children program is a responsibility of state departments of health, not local health departments.

   B. **CORRECT:** Providing education to achieve community health goals is a component of identifying and intervening to meet health needs of the local community, which is a responsibility of local health departments.

   C. **CORRECT:** Funding for local health departments come from local, state and federal monies, therefore; local health departments are responsible for coordinating directives issued from the state level.

   D. INCORRECT: Reporting communicable diseases to the CDC is a responsibility of state departments of health, not local health departments. Local health department report communicable diseases to the state department of health.

   E. INCORRECT: Licensing of registered nurses is incorrect. Licensing of registered nurses is a responsibility of state boards of nursing, not local health departments.

    NCLEX® Connection: Management of Care, Case Management

6. *Using the ATI Active Learning Template: Basic Concept*

A. Underlying Principles

- National health goals:
  - Reduction in per capita domestic water usage
  - Reduction in blood lead levels in children
  - Reduction in indoor allergens
  - Reduction in the number of new schools near highways
  - Increase in schools with policies/practices to promote health and safety
- Environmental health history:
  - What year was your home built?
  - What is you and your partner's current occupation?
  - What recreational activities do your family participate in?
  - Are there any industries or hazardous waste sites nearby?
  - Where does your drinking water come from?

B. Nursing Interventions

- Carbon monoxide is a colorless, odorless gas that is difficult to detect, but is the leading cause of death due to poisoning. Possible sources of carbon monoxide include motor vehicles, gas ranges, vented gas heaters, space heaters, and furnaces. Detectors can be installed within the home to continuously monitor the air for carbon monoxide.

- Keep all potentially toxic agents in the original container and out of the children's reach or in a locked cabinet.

- Be certain to cook meats completely and to wash hands and sanitize countertops after preparing raw meats. Wash raw fruits and vegetables thoroughly before consuming.

- Some potential sources of lead include playground equipment, vinyl mini-blinds, pottery, water, battery casings, certain imported toys, and metal jewelry.

- Teach older children to wash hands when coming in from outside and prior to playing with the newborn.

Ⓝ NCLEX® Connection: Safety and Infection Control, Home Safety

CHAPTER 3   Community Health Program Planning

When reviewing the chapters in this unit, keep in mind the relevant sections of the NCLEX® outline, in particular:

Client Needs: Management of Care	Client Needs: Safety and Infection Control	Client Needs: Health Promotion and Maintenance
› Relevant topics/tasks include:	› Relevant topics/tasks include:	› Relevant topics/tasks include:
» Collaboration with Interprofessional Team	» Accident/Injury Prevention	» Health Promotion/Disease Prevention
› Review the plan of care to ensure continuity across disciplines.	› Identify factors that influence accident/injury prevention.	› Identify risk factors for disease/illness.
» Continuity of Care		
› Follow up on unresolved issues regarding client care.		

Overview

- The role of the community health nurse in community health program planning and evaluation is a collaborative leadership role. The desired outcome is to plan, organize, implement, and evaluate intervention programs that address the specific health needs of the community.

- Community health program planning should reflect the priorities set as a result of analysis of community assessment data. Priorities are established based on the extent of the problem (community members' perception of health needs, percent of population affected by the problem), the relevance of the problem to the public (degree of risk, economic loss), and the estimated impact of intervention (improvement of health outcome, adverse effects).

Community Assessment: Individual, Family, Aggregates

- Community assessment is a comprehensive approach that emphasizes the community as a client.

- Community assessment and diagnosis are the foundation for community-specific program planning.

- Using the nursing process, nurses can determine health needs within the community and assist in developing and implementing strategies to meet those needs. In doing this, it is necessary to expand the assessment, diagnosis, planning, intervention, and evaluation efforts from the individual to the community or aggregate level.

- The community health nurse is a key player in assessing the needs of the community. This role includes:

  - Interacting with community partners serving the community at large.

  - Witnessing the interaction between community programs and the response of the client to the services.

  - Identifying future services based upon the visible needs of community members and population groups.

- Components of a Community Assessment

  - People

    - Demographic – Distribution, mobility, density, census data

    - Biological factors – Health and disease status, genetics, race, age, gender, causes of death

    - Social factors – Occupation, activities, marital status, education, income, crime rates, recreation, industry

    - Cultural factors – Positions, roles, history, values, customs, norms, religion

  - Place or environment

    - Physical factors – Geography, terrain, type of community, location of health services, housing, animal control

    - Environmental factors – Geography, climate, flora, fauna, topography, toxic substances, vectors, pollutants

   ○ Social systems

      ▪ Health systems

      ▪ Economic systems/factors

      ▪ Education systems

      ▪ Religious systems

      ▪ Welfare systems

      ▪ Political systems

      ▪ Recreation systems/factors

      ▪ Legal systems

      ▪ Communication systems/factors

      ▪ Transportation systems

      ▪ Resources and services

Data Collection

- Data collection is a critical community health nursing function. To best identify the health needs of the local community, it is essential to combine several methods of data collection. Relying on only one or two key pieces can result in an incomplete assessment.

INFORMANT INTERVIEWS		
Description	› Direct discussion with community members for the purpose of obtaining ideas and opinions from key informants	
Strengths	› Minimal cost › Participants serving as future supporters › Offer insight into beliefs and attitudes of community members	› Reading/writing of participants not required › Personal interaction may elicit more detailed responses
Limitations	› Built-in bias › Meeting time and place	
COMMUNITY FORUM		
Description	› Open public meeting	
Strengths	› Opportunity for community input › Minimal cost	
Limitations	› Difficulty finding a convenient time and place › Potential to drift from the issue	› Challenging to get adequate participation › Possibility that a less vocal person may be reluctant to speak

SECONDARY DATA	
Description	› Use of existing data (death statistics; birth statistics; census data; mortality, morbidity data; health records; minutes from meetings; prior health surveys) to assess problem
Strengths	› Database of prior concerns/needs of population › Ability to trend health issues over time
Limitations	› Possibility that data may not represent current situation › Can be time-consuming

PARTICIPANT OBSERVATION	
Description	› Observation of formal or informal community activities
Strengths	› Indication of community priorities, environmental profile, and identification of power structures
Limitations	› Bias › Time-consuming › Inability to ask questions of participants

WINDSHIELD SURVEY	
Description	› Descriptive approach that assesses several community components by driving through a community
Strengths	› Provides a descriptive overview of a community
Limitations	› Need for a driver so the nurse can visualize and document the community elements › May be time-consuming › Results based only on visualization and does not include input from community members

FOCUS GROUPS		
Description	› Directed talk with a representative sample	
Strengths	› Possibility of participants being potential supporters › Provides insight into community support › Reading/writing of participants not required	
Limitations	› Possible discussion of irrelevant issues › Challenging to get participants › Requires strong facilitator	› Difficult to ensure that sample is truly representative of the overall community › Time-consuming to transcribe discussion

SURVEYS		
Description	› Specific questions asked in a written format	
Strengths	› Data collected on client population and problems › Random sampling	› Available as written or online format › Contact with participants not required
Limitations	› Low response rate › Expensive › Time-consuming	› Possibility of the collection of superficial data › Requires reading/writing abilities of participants

- Windshield Survey Components
  - People
    - Who is on the street?
    - What is their general appearance (age, dress, well-nourished, obese, frail, unkempt)?
    - What are they doing?
    - What is the origin, ethnicity, or race of the people?
    - How are the different groups (subgroups) residentially located?
    - Is there any evidence of drug abuse, violence, disease, mental illness?
    - Are there any animals or pets in the community?
  - Place
    - Boundaries
      - Where is the community located?
      - What are its boundaries?
      - Are there natural boundaries?
      - Are there man-made boundaries?
    - Location of health services
      - Where are the major health facilities located?
      - What health care facilities are necessary for the community but are not within the community?
    - Natural environment
      - Are there geographic features that may harm the community?
      - Are there plants or animals that could harm or threaten the health of the community?
    - Man-made environment
      - What industries are within the communities?
      - Could these pose a threat to the health of community workers or the community itself?
      - Is there easy access to health care facilities?
      - Are the roads adequate and marked well?
    - Housing
      - Is the housing of acceptable quality?
      - How old are the homes?
      - Are there single or multifamily dwellings?
      - Is the housing in good repair or disrepair?
      - Is there vacant housing?

- Social systems
  - Are there social services, clinics, hospitals, dentists, and health care providers available within the community?
  - Are there ample schools within the community? Are they in good repair or disrepair?
  - Are there parks or areas for recreation?
  - What places of worship are within the community?
  - What services are provided by local religious groups, schools, community centers, and activity or recreation centers?
  - Is there public transportation?
  - What grocery stores or other stores are within the community?
  - Is public protection evident (police, fire, EMS services, animal control)?

Analysis of Community Assessment Data

- The community health nurse plays an active role in assessment, data interpretation, and problem identification. Steps in analysis of community assessment data include:
  - Gathering collected data into a composite database.
  - Assessing completeness of data.
  - Identifying and generating missing data.
  - Synthesizing data and identifying themes.
  - Identifying community needs and problems.
  - Identifying community strengths and resources.
- Problem analysis is completed for each identified problem. Frequently, work groups are formed to examine individual problems and develop solutions.

Community Health Diagnoses

- Problems identified by community assessments are often stated as community health diagnoses.
- Community nursing diagnoses incorporate information from the community assessment, general nursing knowledge, and epidemiological concepts (especially the concept of risk in a population).
- Community nursing diagnoses often are written in the following format:
  - Risk of (specific problem or risk in the community) among (the specific population that is affected by the problem or risk) related to (strengths and weaknesses in the community that influence the problem or risk).

Community Health Program Planning, Development, and Management

PREPLANNING	
Description	› Brainstorm ideas.
Activities	› Gain entry into community and establish trust. › Obtain community awareness, support, and involvement. › Coordinate collaborations that have similar interests in addressing identified problems.

ASSESSMENT	
Description	› Collect data about the community and its members.
Activities	› Complete a needs assessment and identify community strengths and weaknesses. › Assess the availability of community resources. › Evaluate secondary health data.

DIAGNOSIS	
Description	› Identify and prioritize health needs of the community.

Activities	› Analyze data to determine health needs.
	› Work with community members, local health professionals and administrators to develop priorities and establish outcomes.
	› In setting priorities among identified community problems, consider the following:
	  » Community awareness of the problem
	  » Community readiness to acknowledge and address the problem
	  » Available expertise/fiscal resources
	  » Severity of the problem
	  » Amount of time needed for problem resolution

PLANNING	
Description	› Develop interventions to meet identified outcomes.
Activities	› Determine possible solutions to meet the health need and select the best option. › Establish goals and objectives for the selected solution. » Objectives are behaviorally stated, measurable, and include a target date for achievement. › Select strategies/interventions to meet the objectives. › Plan a logical sequence for interventions by establishing a timetable. › Identify who will assume responsibility for each intervention. › Determine available and needed resources to implement interventions. › Assess the personnel needed and any special training they may require for screening or providing education. › Determine funding opportunities for needed interventions and develop a budget. › Plan for program evaluation.

IMPLEMENTATION	
Description	› Carry out the plan.
Activities	› Initiate interventions to achieve goals and objectives according to program plan. › Monitor the intervention process and the response of the community in terms of its values, needs, and perceptions.

EVALUATION	
Description	› Examine the success of the interventions.
Activities	› Evaluate strengths and weaknesses of the program. › Determine achievement of desired outcomes. › Examine the adequacy, efficiency, appropriateness, and cost benefit of the program. › Recommend and implement modifications to better meet the needs of the community. › Share findings and recommendations with community members and stakeholders. › Ongoing evaluation is necessary in order to ensure program success and meet the changing needs of the community.

Strategies for and Barriers to Implementing Community Health Programs

HELPFUL STRATEGIES	BARRIERS
› Thorough assessment	› Inadequate assessment
› Accurate interpretation of data	› Inadequate or misconstrued data
› Collaboration with community partners	› No involvement with community partners
› Effective communication patterns	› Impaired communication
› Sufficient resources	› Inadequate resources
› Logical planning	› Lack of planning
› Skilled leadership	› Poor leadership

APPLICATION EXERCISES

1. A nurse is preparing to conduct a windshield survey. Which of the following data should the nurse collect as a component of this assessment? (Select all that apply.)

_____ A. Ethnicity of community members

_____ B. Individuals who hold power within the community

_____ C. Natural community boundaries

_____ D. Prevalence of disease

_____ E. Presence of public protection

2. A nurse is completing a needs assessment and beginning analysis of data. Which of the following actions should the nurse take first?

A. Determine health patterns within collected data.

B. Compile collected data into a database.

C. Ensure data collection is complete.

D. Identify health needs of the local community.

3. A nurse is planning a community health program. Which of the following should the nurse include as part of the evaluation plan?

A. Determine availability of resources to initiate the plan.

B. Gain approval for the program from local leaders.

C. Establish a timeline for implementation of interventions.

D. Compare program impact to similar programs.

4. A nurse is conducting a community assessment. Which of the following data collection methods is the nurse using when having direct conversations with individual members of the community?

A. Key informant interviews

B. Participant observation

C. Focus groups

D. Health surveys

5. A nurse is collecting data to identify health needs in the local community. Which of the following are examples of secondary data the nurse should review? (Select all that apply.)

_____ A. Birth statistics

_____ B. Previous health survey results

_____ C. Windshield survey

_____ D. Community forum

_____ E. Health records

6. A nurse collects the following data during a community assessment:

> Low crime rate
> Curbside garbage pick-up
> Increased incidence of low infant birth weight

> Small amount of litter along the road
> Public transportation that operates 24 hr a day, 7 days a week

> Older playground equipment in need of repair.
> High prevalence of diabetes mellitus
> Recreational trails that are in need of maintenance.

Using the ATI Active Learning Template: Basic Concept, complete this item to include the following:

A. Underlying Principles: Identify possible methods of collecting the data resulting from the nurse's community assessment.

B. Nursing Interventions:

- Name one action the nurse should take as part of the diagnosis phase of program development.

- Name three actions the nurse should take as part of the planning phase of program development.

APPLICATION EXERCISES KEY

1. A. **CORRECT:** The nurse should identify the ethnicity of the people visible in the community as a component a windshield survey.

    B. INCORRECT: Individuals who hold power are identified through formal and informal observations of community activities, as a participant observer.

    C. **CORRECT:** The nurse should identify natural community boundaries as a component a windshield survey.

    D. INCORRECT: Prevalence of disease is incorrect. Disease prevalence is a component of secondary data and is identified through morbidity rates of the community.

    E. **CORRECT:** The nurse should identify the presence of public protection, such as police, fire, and animal control, as a component a windshield survey.

     NCLEX® Connection: Psychosocial Integrity, Stress Management

2. A. INCORRECT: This is not the first action the nurse should take. In order to determine health patterns within collected data the nurse must take another action first.

    B. **CORRECT:** This is the first action the nurse should take. In order to adequately and appropriately analyze collected data the nurse must first compile collected data into a database.

    C. INCORRECT: This is not the first action the nurse should take. In order to ensure data collection is complete the nurse must take another action first.

    D. INCORRECT: This is not the first action the nurse should take. In order to identify health needs of the local community the nurse must take another action first.

     NCLEX® Connection: Management of Care, Establishing Priorities

3. A. INCORRECT: The nurse should not include determining availability of resources to initiate the program as part of the evaluation plan; this should be done during the assessment phase. However, when evaluating sustainability of the program, the nurse should determine whether resources are available for continuing the program.

   B. INCORRECT: The nurse should not include gaining approval for the program from local leaders as part of the evaluation plan. This approval should take place as part of the preplanning phase because plans for the program should not move forward without adequate community support.

   C. INCORRECT: The nurse should not include establishing a timeline for implementation of interventions as part of the evaluation plan. Timeline development should occur after determining and selecting the best strategies for meeting the program's goals and objectives.

   D. **CORRECT:** The nurse should include comparing program impact to similar programs as part of the evaluation plan. This comparison assists with determining the efficiency of the program.

   N NCLEX® Connection: Health Promotion and Maintenance, Health Promotion/Disease Prevention

4. A. **CORRECT:** Informant interviews are direct conversations with individual community members for the purpose of obtaining ideas and opinions.

   B. INCORRECT: Participant observation is observing formal or informal community activities and does not involve direct conversations with individual community members.

   C. INCORRECT: Focus groups are directed talks with a representative sample of a community, and do not involve direct conversations with individual community members.

   D. INCORRECT: Surveys are specific questions asked in a written format and do not involve direct conversations with individual community members.

   N NCLEX® Connection: Health Promotion and Maintenance, Health Promotion/Disease Prevention

5. A. **CORRECT:** Birth statistics are an example of secondary data the nurse should review.

   B. **CORRECT:** Previous health survey results are an example of secondary data the nurse should review.

   C. INCORRECT: Windshield surveys are a method of collecting direct data.

   D. INCORRECT: Community forums are a method of collecting direct data.

   E. **CORRECT:** Health records are an example of secondary data the nurse should review.

   N NCLEX® Connection: Health Promotion and Maintenance, Health Promotion/Disease Prevention

6. *Using the ATI Active Learning Template: Basic Concept*

A. Underlying Principles
- Data collection methods
  - Curbside garbage pick-up – windshield survey; key informant interview; focus group
  - Increased incidence of low infant birth weight – secondary data from health statistics
  - Small amount of litter along the road – windshield survey
  - Public transportation that operates 24 hr a day, 7 days a week – windshield survey; key informant interview
  - Older playground equipment in need of repair – windshield survey; key informant interview; focus group
  - High prevalence of diabetes mellitus – secondary data from health statistics
  - Recreational trails that are in need of maintenance – windshield survey; key informant interview; focus group

B. Nursing Interventions
- Diagnosis phase
  - Analyze collected data to determine health needs within the local community.
  - Work with community members, local health professionals and administrators to develop priorities and establish outcomes for identified health needs.
- Planning phase
  - Determine possible solutions to meet health needs of the community and select the best option.
  - Establish goals and objectives for the selected solution.
  - Select strategies/interventions to meet the objectives.
  - Establish a timeline for implementation of interventions.
  - Identify resources that are available, and resources that are needed, to implement strategies.
  - Determine funding opportunities for needed interventions and develop a budget.
  - Plan for program evaluation.

Ⓝ NCLEX® Connection: Health Promotion and Maintenance, Health Promotion/Disease Prevention

CHAPTER 4   Practice Settings and Aggregates

NCLEX® CONNECTIONS

When reviewing the chapters in this unit, keep in mind the relevant sections of the NCLEX® outline, in particular:

Client Needs: Safety and Infection Control

› Relevant topics/tasks include:

» Accident/Injury Prevention

› Identify deficits that may impede client safety.

» Handling Hazardous and Infectious Materials

› Follow procedures for handling biohazardous materials.

» Standard Precautions/ Transmission-Based Precautions/Surgical Asepsis

› Follow correct policy and procedures when reporting a client with a communicable disease.

Client Needs: Health Promotion and Maintenance

› Relevant topics/tasks include:

» Health Promotion/Disease Prevention

› Assess and teach clients about health risks based on family, population, and/or community characteristics.

» High-Risk Behaviors

› Assist the client to identify behaviors/risks that may impact health.

Client Needs: Psychosocial Integrity

› Relevant topics/tasks include:

» End of Life Care

› Provide end of life care and education to clients.

» Religious and Spiritual Influences on Health

› Assess psychosocial, spiritual, and occupational factors affecting care and plan interventions, as appropriate.

chapter 4

Overview

- Community health nurses practice in diverse settings.
- Community health nurses practice as:
  - Home health nurses
  - Hospice nurses
  - Occupational health nurses
  - Parish nurses
  - School nurses
  - Case managers
- Aggregates receive services from community health nurses.
  - Individuals from infancy to death
  - Families
  - Groups within the community
- It is important to be aware of health disparities of each group and to minimize those disparities when possible.

Practice Settings

- Home Health Nurse
  - Community health nurses provide health care services to clients where they reside. This includes traditional homes, assisted living facilities, and nursing homes.
  - Working as part of an interprofessional team is essential to providing holistic care.
    - Nurses, physical therapists, occupational therapists, home health aides, social workers, and dietitians may be part of the interprofessional care provided in the home.
    - These services are prescribed by a primary care provider and usually are coordinated by a nurse.
  - The home health nurse functions as educator, provider of skilled nursing interventions, and coordinator of care.
    - Many clients leave the hospital in just a few days and are still very ill.
    - These clients and their family members need skilled services and education about the disease process, prescribed medications, and future implications of their illnesses.

- Home health nurses provide a variety of skilled services, including the following:
  - Skilled assessment
  - Wound care
  - Laboratory draws
  - Medication education and administration
  - Parenteral nutrition
  - IV fluids and medication
  - Central line care
  - Urinary catheter insertion and maintenance
  - Coordination/supervision of various other participants in health services
- The home health nurse must evaluate the living environment for safety, paying close attention to nonsecure rugs, electrical outlets, and extension cords; the use of oxygen; safety devices in the bathroom; and other potential environmental hazards.
  - Older adults are at a particular risk for falls.
  - Nurses should ask the following questions:
    - Does the client have food in the house to eat?
    - Is there help with household activities?
    - Does the client live alone?
    - Who is the client's support system?
    - Is the client able to set up and dispense his own medication?
    - Does the client have access to health care?
- Home health nurses provide follow-up care after an acute hospital stay. Therefore, they must educate the client and the family regarding complications or adverse reactions.
  - These instructions may include when to contact the agency, the emergency room, or the provider. Information and resources for families and clients can provide support in dealing with illness.
- Providing education encourages clients to be independent and to be involved in their own care. It also allows families to be involved in the care and decision-making regarding their family members.

- Hospice Nurse
  - Hospice care focuses on enhancing the quality of life through the provision of palliative care, supporting the client and family through the dying process, and providing bereavement support to the family following the client's death.
  - Hospice care is provided in a variety of settings, including the home, hospice centers, hospitals, and long-term care settings.
  - Hospice care is a comprehensive care delivery system for clients who are terminally ill. Further medical care aimed toward a cure is stopped. The focus becomes relief of pain and suffering, as well as enhancing quality of life.
  - Care is provided for the client and the client's entire family.

- Hospice care uses an interprofessional approach.
- Controlling symptoms is a priority.
- Hospice care services are directed by the provider and managed by the nurse.
- Volunteers are used for nonmedical care.
- Postmortem bereavement services are offered for the family.
- Helping the family transition from an expectation of recovery to acceptance of death is an important aspect of providing hospice care. The hospice nurse may continue to work with the family for up to 1 year following the death of the client.

- Occupational Health Nurse
  - All work environments have associated risks. Health care in the workplace seeks to both promote health and prevent occupational illness and injury. Through improvement and maintenance of health, workplace expenditures are decreased by less sick time use, fewer workers compensation claims, and decreased use of group health coverage.
  - Nurses function in numerous roles within workplace settings and are challenged to provide cost-effective and high-quality care. In this effort it is essential for the occupational health nurse to develop partnerships with workplace administration, industrial hygienists, safety specialists, occupational medicine physicians, human resource departments, union representatives, and health insurance agencies.
  - The occupational health nurse works toward the health and safety of workers.
    - Assessing risks for work-related illness and injury.
    - Planning and delivering health and safety services in the workplace.
    - Facilitating health promotion activities that lead to a more productive workforce.
  - This autonomous specialty entails making independent nursing judgments when providing care to the workforce aggregate.
  - In assessing risk for work-related illness and injury, the nurse should keep in mind the following factors affecting susceptibility to illness and injury:
    - Host factors
      - Worker characteristics, such as job inexperience, age, and pregnancy.
    - Agent factors
      - Biological agents (viruses, bacteria, fungi, blood-borne, airborne pathogens)
      - Chemical agents (asbestos, smoke)
      - Mechanical agents (musculoskeletal or other strains from repetitive motions, poor workstation-worker fit, lifting heavy loads)
      - Physical agents (temperature extremes, vibrations, noise, radiation, lighting)
      - Psychological agents (threats to psychological or social well-being resulting in work-related stress, burnout, violence)
    - Environmental factors
      - Physical factors (heat, odor, ventilation, pollution)
      - Social factors (sanitation, overcrowding)
      - Psychological factors (addictions, stress)

○ Occupational health nurses' roles and responsibilities include the following:

- Primary prevention – Teaching good nutrition and knowledge of health hazards, and providing information on immunizations, and use of protective equipment.

- Secondary prevention – Identifying workplace hazards, early detection through health surveillance and screening, prompt treatment, counseling and referral, and prevention of further limitations.

- Tertiary prevention – Restoration of health through rehabilitation strategies and limited-duty programs.

○ An occupational health history provides the framework for a nurse to begin to assess a worker for possible exposure to health hazards.

- The goal is to identify agents and host factors that place the worker at risk, identify ways to eliminate or minimize exposure, and prevent potential health problems.

- Information elicited should include the following:

  □ Current and past jobs

  □ Current and past exposure to specific agents and any relationship of current symptoms to work activities

  □ Any precipitating factors, such as underlying illness, previous injuries, and healthy or unhealthy habits

○ A work site walk-through or survey is also part of a workplace assessment. Focus should be given to the following:

- Observation of work processes and materials

- Job requirements

- Actual and potential hazards

- Employee work practices (hygiene, waste disposal, housekeeping)

- Incidence/prevalence of work-related illness/injuries

- Control strategies to eliminate exposures

○ Control strategies are designed to reduce future exposures based upon results from investigations into work-related illness/injury. Control strategies often include the following:

- Engineering

- Altering work practices

- Providing personal protective equipment and education to prevent future injuries

- Workplace monitoring

- Health screening

- Employee-assistance programs

- Job-task analysis

- Design, risk management, and emergency preparedness

- ○ Protection from violence

  - Work can be frustrating and can contribute to stress, resulting in aggression and violence against others.

  - Being aware of jobs that are repetitive, boring, or physically and psychologically draining can help to identify workers who may feel tired, angry, and generally inadequate.

  - Nurses can refer such workers to employee-assistance programs that provide confidential counseling and referrals to other professional services if needed.

- ○ Protection from work-related injuries from falls, environmental hazards, and burns

  - Nurses can use research and trend analysis to improve working conditions by eliminating or minimizing hazards and potential problems.

  - Additional strategies include:

    - □ Providing safety and health education programs to workers.

    - □ Developing health policy focused on ensuring effective employee health and safety.

    - □ Designing strategies to prevent work-related accidents/injuries.

    - □ Keeping abreast of Occupational Health and Safety Administration (OSHA) standards and resource programs.

    - □ Working to influence legislation aimed at workers/workplace health protection.

- ○ Occupational Health and Legislation

  - The Occupational Safety and Health Act of 1970

    - □ Occupational Health and Safety Administration (OSHA) – Develops and enforces workplace health regulations to protect the safety and health of workers.

    - □ National Advisory Committee on Occupational Safety and Health (NACOSH) – Gathers and disseminates data on the incidence and prevalence of occupational illness and injury. This agency is also responsible for prevention education related to occupational injury and illness, as well as determining hazards associated with new workplace technologies.

  - Workers Compensation Acts – State-level legislation that regulates financial compensation to workers suffering from injuries or illness resulting from the workplace.

- • Faith Community Nurse

  - ○ The faith community nurse works with a group of clients who share common faith traditions. Most religions have practices that are important to health and healing, and many follow specific practices when caring for an ill or dying member.

  - ○ Members of faith communities represent the entire lifespan and all family types. This offers nurses the opportunity to work with a diverse population within the same setting.

  - ○ Caring and spirituality are central among faith-based organizations.

    - CIRCLE Model of Spiritual Care

      - □ Caring

      - □ Intuition

      - □ Respect for religious beliefs and practices

      - □ Caution

      - □ Listening

      - □ Emotional support

- ○ Missionary Nurse

  - Missionary nursing seeks to promote health and prevent disease by meeting spiritual, physical, and emotional needs of people across the globe. These nurses may be career missionaries, or may serve as short-term, volunteer, or part-time missionaries.

  - Cultural and language barriers often affect the provision of care. Collaboration within the community is essential in meeting goals.

- ○ Parish Nurse

  - Parish nurses promote the health and wellness of populations of faith communities. The population often includes church members and individuals and groups in the geographical community.

  - Parish nurses work closely with pastoral care staff, professional health care members, and lay volunteers to provide a holistic approach to healing (body, mind, and spirit).

  - Functions of the parish nurse

    - □ Personal health counseling (health-risk appraisals, spiritual assessments, support for numerous acute and chronic, actual and potential health problems)

    - □ Health education (available resources, classes, individual and group teaching)

    - □ Liaison between faith community and local resources

    - □ Facilitating support groups

    - □ Spiritual support (help identify spiritual strengths for coping)

- School Nurse

  - ○ School nursing encompasses many roles.

    - Case manager: coordinates comprehensive services for children who have complex health needs.

    - Community outreach: strives to meet the needs of all school-age children by cooperative planning and collaboration between the educational system and other community agencies.

    - Consultant: assists students, families, and personnel in information gathering and decision-making about a variety of health needs and resources.

    - Counselor: supports students on a wide variety of health needs.

    - Direct caregiver: provides nursing care to ill or injured children at school.

    - Health educator: helps prepare children, families, school personnel, and the community to make well-informed health decisions.

    - Researcher: contributes to the base of knowledge for school health and educational needs.

LEVELS OF PREVENTION IN SCHOOL NURSING	
ASSESSMENTS	**EXAMPLES OF NURSING INTERVENTIONS**
Primary prevention	
› Assess the knowledge base regarding health issues.	› Teach health promotion practices: » Hand hygiene and tooth-brushing » Healthy food choices » Injury prevention, including bike and water safety » Substance dependency prevention
› Assess the immunization status of all children.	› Maintain current records of required immunizations.
Secondary prevention	
› Assess children who become ill or injured at school.	› Provide care to children who have » Headaches » Stomach pain » Injuries that occur at school
› Assess all children, faculty, and staff during emergencies.	› Provide emergency care such as first aid and CPR. › The school clinic should have commonly needed supplies.
› Perform screening for early detection of disease.	› Screenings » Vision and hearing » Height and weight » Oral health » Scoliosis » Infestations (lice) » General physical examinations
› Assess children to detect child abuse or neglect.	› The school nurse is required by state law to officially report all suspected cases of child abuse/neglect.
› Assess children for evidence of mental illness, suicide, and violence.	› Identify children at risk.
Tertiary prevention	
› Assess children with disabilities.	› Participate in developing the individual education plan (IEP) for children with disabilities. › Work with child/family to develop and achieve long-term outcomes.
› Assess children with long-term health needs at school.	› Provide nursing care for children with disorders, including asthma, diabetes mellitus, and cystic fibrosis. › Administer medication per provider's prescription. › The prescribed medication should be in the original bottle and be stored in a secure place. › Written consent by the parents is required. › Provide care to children who have specific health needs, including: » Urinary catheterizations » Dressing changes » IV line monitoring

COMPONENTS OF COORDINATED SCHOOL HEALTH PROGRAMS	
Health education	› Inclusion of health concepts in courses of study for children in pre-K through grade 12
Physical education	› Promoting physical activity in school
Health services	› Providing health services in school by qualified professionals (nurses, physicians, dentists, allied health professionals)
Nutrition services	› Providing access to meals that accommodate the health and nutrition needs of all children
Counseling, psychological, and social services	› Services that improve the mental, emotional, and social health of students, as well as the overall school
Promotion of a healthy and safe school environment	› Reducing tobacco use and violence in schools
Health promotion for staff	› Activities that encourage health promotion and disease prevention behaviors among the school's faculty and staff
Facilitation of family/community involvement	› Promoting collaboration between the school, parents/caregivers, and community resources

Aggregates of the Community

- Children (Birth to 12 Years) and Adolescents
  - Health concerns/leading causes of death
    - Children
      - Perinatal conditions/congenital anomalies
      - Sudden Infant Death Syndrome (SIDS)
      - Motor vehicle/other unintentional injuries
    - Adolescents
      - Motor vehicle/other unintentional injuries
      - Homicide
      - Suicide
  - Screening/preventive services
    - Children
      - Height/weight
      - Vision and hearing
      - At birth – hemoglobinopathy, phenylalanine level, T4, and TSH
      - Immunization status – check the Centers for Disease Control and Prevention (CDC) website, www.cdc.gov, for current administration schedules
      - Cholesterol and triglyceride levels
      - Dental health

- Adolescents
  - Height/weight
  - Dental health
  - Rubella serology/vaccination history (females)
  - Substance use disorders, including tobacco
  - Immunization status (www.cdc.gov)
  - Mental health screenings
  - Cholesterol and triglyceride levels
  - Vision and hearing
- National health goals
  - Children
    - Reductions in
      - Dental caries
      - Obesity
      - Exposure to secondhand smoke
    - Increases in
      - Newborn blood spot screenings and follow-up testing
      - Access to a medical home
      - Schools that require health education
      - Childhood immunizations
      - Use of child safety restraints
      - Physical activity
  - Adolescents
    - Reductions in
      - Violent crimes
      - Initiation of tobacco use
      - Obesity
      - Inappropriate weight gain
    - Increases in
      - Schools with a breakfast program
      - Participation in extracurricular activities
      - Wellness checkups within prior 12 months
      - Physical activity

- ○ Community education
  - ■ Children
    - □ Anticipatory guidance
    - □ Breastfeeding
    - □ Sleeping positions
    - □ Nutrition
    - □ Physical activity
    - □ Substance use disorders
    - □ Dental hygiene/health
    - □ Skin protection
    - □ Injury prevention including car, fire, and water safety; helmet use; poison control; and CPR training
  - ■ Adolescents
    - □ Anticipatory guidance
    - □ Substance use disorders
    - □ Sexual behavior
    - □ Nutrition, especially calcium intake for females
    - □ Physical activity
    - □ Skin protection
    - □ Injury prevention including car, fire, and firearm safety
- • Women
  - ○ Health concerns/leading causes of death
    - ■ Reproductive health
      - □ Childbearing
      - □ Menopause
      - □ Osteoporosis
    - ■ Heart disease
    - ■ Diabetes mellitus
    - ■ Malignant neoplasm (breast, cervical, ovarian, colorectal)
  - ○ Screening/Preventive Services
    - ■ Height/weight
    - ■ Blood pressure
    - ■ Cholesterol (ages 45 to 65)
    - ■ Dental health
    - ■ Pap smear test
    - ■ Mammogram/clinical breast exam
    - ■ Fecal occult blood test/sigmoidoscopy (≥ 50 years)
    - ■ Rubella serology/vaccination history (childbearing years)

- Immunization status – check the CDC website, www.cdc.gov, for current administration schedules
- Diabetes mellitus
- HIV
- Skin cancer

- ○ National Health Goals
  - Reductions in
    - □ Diseases involving bone, such as osteoporosis
    - □ Death from cancer such as breast, ovarian, and cervical
    - □ Sexual violence
  - Increases in
    - □ Number of planned pregnancies versus unplanned
    - □ Those who receive early and adequate prenatal care
    - □ The number of mothers who breastfeed
    - □ Ability to identify warning signs of a heart attack and stroke
- ○ Community Education
  - Nutrition
  - STI prevention
  - Substance use disorders
  - Breast self-examination
  - Skin protection
  - HIV prevention
  - Injury prevention including car, fire safety, and violence
- Men
  - ○ Health concerns/leading causes of death
    - Heart disease
    - Malignant neoplasm (prostate, testicular, skin, colorectal)
    - Unintentional injuries
    - Lung disease
    - Liver disease
  - ○ Screening/Preventive Services
    - Height/weight
    - Blood pressure
    - Dental health
    - Digital rectal exam
    - Fecal occult blood test/sigmoidoscopy (≥ 50 years)
    - Immunization status – check the CDC website, www.cdc.gov, for current administration schedules
    - Diabetes mellitus

- HIV
- Skin cancer
- Cholesterol (ages 45 to 65 years)
- National Health Goals
  - Reductions in
    - Death from cancer specific to men, such as prostate
    - Incidence of HIV and AIDS
    - Fatal and nonfatal injuries
  - Increases in
    - Participation in aerobic and muscle-strengthening activities
    - Ability to identify warning signs of a heart attack and stroke
- Community Education
  - Nutrition
  - Self-testicular exam
  - Skin protection
  - Substance use disorders
  - HIV prevention
  - Injury prevention including car, fire and firearm safety, and violence
- Older Adults
  - Health concerns/leading causes of death
    - Heart disease
    - Malignant neoplasm
    - Cerebrovascular disease
    - Chronic obstructive pulmonary disease
    - Pneumonia and influenza
    - Substance use and misuse
  - Screening/Preventive Services
    - Blood pressure
    - Height/weight
    - Dental health
    - Fecal occult blood test/sigmoidoscopy
    - Mammogram/clinical breast exam (women)
    - Pap smear test (women)
    - Vision
    - Hearing
    - Substance use
    - Immunization status (pneumococcal, influenza) – check the CDC website, www.cdc.gov, for current administration schedules

- Functional assessment (self-care abilities)
- Medication history
- Osteoporosis
- Diabetes mellitus
- Skin cancer

- ○ National Health Goals
  - Reductions in
    - □ Adults who have musculoskeletal concerns
    - □ Older adults who have mental health concerns
    - □ Hospitalizations due to heart failure
    - □ Substance use in the older adult
    - □ Sensory concerns such as hearing loss and cataracts
    - □ Hip fractures among older adults
    - □ Fall-related deaths
  - Increases in
    - □ Screenings for colorectal cancer
    - □ Participation in organized health promotion activities
    - □ Public reporting of elder maltreatment
    - □ Older adults who maintain an active lifestyle
- ○ Community Education
  - Substance use disorders
  - Nutrition
  - Exercise
  - Dental health
  - Sexual behavior
  - Injury prevention
    - □ Car and fire safety
    - □ Fall prevention
    - □ Violence
- Families
  - ○ The family as client is basic to community-oriented nursing practice. Community health nurses have a significant role to play in promoting healthy families.
  - ○ Community health nurses must engage in community assessment, planning, development, and evaluation activities that are focused on family issues.
  - ○ Home visits provide community health nurses with the opportunity to observe the home environment and to identify barriers and supports to health-risk reduction.
  - ○ Family crisis occurs when a family is not able to cope with an event. The family's resources are inadequate for the demands of the situation.

- ○ Transitions are times of risk for families.
  - ▪ Transitions include birth or adoption of a child, death of a family member, child moving out of the home, marriage of a child, major illness, divorce, and loss of the main family income.
  - ▪ These transitions require families to change behaviors, make new decisions, reallocate family roles, learn new skills, and learn to use new resources.
- ○ Characteristics of healthy families
  - ▪ Members communicate well and listen to each other.
  - ▪ There is affirmation and support for all members.
  - ▪ Members teach respect for others.
  - ▪ There is a sense of trust.
  - ▪ Members play and share humor together.
  - ▪ Members interact with one another.
  - ▪ There is a shared sense of responsibility.
  - ▪ There are traditions and rituals.
  - ▪ Members seek help for their problems.
- ○ Family health risk appraisal
  - ▪ Biological health risk assessment
    - □ Genograms are used to gather basic information about the family, relationships within the family, and health and illness patterns.
    - □ Repetitions of diseases with a genetic component (cancer, heart disease, diabetes mellitus) can be identified.
  - ▪ Environmental risk: Ecomaps are used to identify family interactions with other groups and organizations. Information about the family's support network and social risk is gathered.
  - ▪ Behavioral risk: Information is gathered about the family's health behavior, including health values, health habits, and health risk perceptions.
- ○ National Health Goals
  - ▪ Reductions in
    - □ Barriers to access
    - □ Allergic content within the home
    - □ Families that are unable to have a child or maintain a pregnancy
    - □ Passive smoke exposure
    - □ Household hunger
  - ▪ Increases in
    - □ Health education provided by an agency (Head Start, school system, college, places of employment, health departments)
    - □ Home testing for radon
    - □ Health insurance coverage
    - □ Individuals who have a usual primary care provider

APPLICATION EXERCISES

1. A nurse is talking to a client who asks for additional information about hospice. Which of the following is an appropriate statement by the nurse?

    A. "Clients who require skilled nursing care at home qualify for hospice care."

    B. "One function of hospice is to provide teaching to clients about life-sustaining measures."

    C. "Hospice assists clients to develop the skills needed to care for themselves independently."

    D. "A component of hospice care is to control the client's symptoms."

2. An occupational health nurse is consulting with senior management of a local industrial facility. When discussing work-related illness and injury, the nurse should include which of the following as physical agents? (Select all that apply.)

    _____ A. Noise

    _____ B. Age

    _____ C. Lighting

    _____ D. Viruses

    _____ E. Stress

3. A newly hired occupational health nurse at an industrial facility is performing an initial workplace assessment. Which of the following should the nurse determine when conducting a work site survey?

    A. Work practices of employees

    B. Past exposure to specific agents

    C. Past jobs of individual employees

    D. Length of time working in current role

4. A school nurse is scheduling visits with a physical therapist for a child who has cerebral palsy. In which of the following roles is the nurse functioning?

    A. Direct caregiver

    B. Consultant

    C. Case manager

    D. Counselor

5. A school nurse is planning health promotion and disease prevention activities for the upcoming school year. In which of the following situations is the nurse planning a secondary prevention strategy?

    A. Placing posters with images of appropriate hand hygiene near restrooms

    B. Routinely checking students for pediculosis throughout the school year

    C. Implementing age-appropriate injury prevention programs for each grade level

    D. Working with a dietician to determine carbohydrate counts for students who have diabetes mellitus

6. A nurse is developing programs to promote the health of families in the local community. Using the ATI Active Learning Template: Basic Concept, complete this item to include the following:

    A. Related Content: Three characteristics of families.

    B. Underlying Principles:

        • Two times families experience transition.

        • Two national health goals that apply to families.

    C. Nursing Interventions: Two strategies to improve the health of families.

APPLICATION EXERCISES KEY

1. A. INCORRECT: Clients who require skilled nursing care at home qualify for home health.

    B. INCORRECT: Home health may provide teaching to clients about life-sustaining measures, but this is not a function of hospice.

    C. INCORRECT: Home health assists clients to develop the skills needed to care for themselves independently.

    D. **CORRECT:** Controlling the client's symptoms is a component of hospice care.

     NCLEX® Connection: Psychosocial Integrity, End of Life Care

2. A. **CORRECT:** The nurse manager should include noise as a physical agent when discussing work-related illness and injury.

    B. INCORRECT: The nurse manager should include age as a host factor when discussing work-related illness and injury.

    C. **CORRECT:** The nurse manager should include lighting as a physical agent when discussing work-related illness and injury.

    D. INCORRECT: The nurse manager should include viruses as a biological agent when discussing work-related illness and injury.

    E. INCORRECT: The nurse manager should include stress as an outcome of psychological agents when discussing work-related illness and injury.

     NCLEX® Connection: Psychosocial Integrity, Stress Management

3. A. **CORRECT:** The nurse should determine the work practices of employees when conducting a work site survey.

    B. INCORRECT: The nurse should determine past exposure to specific agents when conducting an occupational health history on individual workers, not a work site survey.

    C. INCORRECT: The nurse should determine past jobs of individual employees when conducting an occupational health history on individual workers, not a work site survey.

    D. INCORRECT: The nurse should determine the length of time working in current role when conducting an occupational health history on individual workers, not a work site survey.

     NCLEX® Connection: Health Promotion and Maintenance, Health Promotion/Disease Prevention

4.   A. INCORRECT: The nurse is not functioning in the role of direct caregiver. As a direct caregiver, a nurse provides illness or injury care to children at school.

     B. INCORRECT: The nurse is not functioning in the role of consultant. As a consultant, a nurse provides information to families, administrators, teachers, and parent-teacher groups to encourage decisions that promote the health of the students.

     C. **CORRECT:** The nurse is functioning in the role of case manager. As a case manager, the nurse coordinates comprehensive services for students with complex health needs.

     D. INCORRECT: The nurse is not functioning in the role of counselor. As a counselor, a nurse develops a trusting relationship with students and provides support on issues affecting their lives.

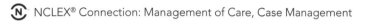 NCLEX® Connection: Management of Care, Case Management

5.   A. INCORRECT: Placing posters with images of appropriate hand hygiene near restrooms is a primary prevention strategy.

     B. **CORRECT:** Routinely checking students for pediculosis throughout the school year is a secondary prevention strategy.

     C. INCORRECT: Implementing age-appropriate injury prevention programs for each grade level is a primary prevention activity.

     D. INCORRECT: Working with the dietitian to determine carbohydrate counts for students with diabetes is a tertiary prevention activity.

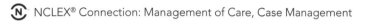 NCLEX® Connection: Health Promotion and Maintenance, Health Screening

6. *Using the ATI Active Learning Template: Basic Concept*

A. Related Content

- Family characteristics

  - Members communicate well and listen to each other.

  - There is affirmation and support for all members.

  - Members teach respect for others.

  - There is a sense of trust.

  - Members play and share humor together.

  - Members interact with one another.

  - There is a shared sense of responsibility.

  - There are traditions and rituals.

  - Members seek help for their problems.

B. Underlying Principles

- Times of transition

  - Birth of a child

  - Adoption of a child

  - Death of a family member

  - Child moving from the home

  - Child getting married

  - Major illness of a family member

  - Divorce of a family member

  - Loss of the main source of family income

- National Health Goals

  - Reductions in

    - Barriers to access

    - Allergic content within the home

    - Families that are unable to have a child or maintain a pregnancy

    - Exposure to secondhand smoke

    - Household hunger

  - Increases in

    - Health education provided by an agency

    - Home testing for radon

    - Health insurance coverage

    - Individuals with a usual primary care provider

C. Nursing Interventions

- Strategies to improve health of families

  - Identify barriers and supports to health-risk reduction.

  - Assess safety during home visits.

  - Identify and coordinate needed community resource referrals.

  - Perform biological health risk assessments.

  - Assess for environmental and behavioral risks.

NCLEX® Connection: Health Promotion and Maintenance, Health Promotion/Disease Prevention

CHAPTER 5 Care of Special Populations

chapter 5

Overview

- Community health nurses care for many individuals who are members of special populations. These vulnerable populations include individuals who are subject to issues such as:
  - Violence
  - Substance use disorders
  - Mental health issues/illnesses
  - Homelessness
  - Rural and migrant health
- These individuals have difficulty accessing health care.
- Other factors that affect these individuals include the following:
  - Poverty
  - Difficulty accessing health care
  - Poor self-esteem
  - Young or advanced age
  - Chronic stress
  - Environmental factors
- National health goals to address for vulnerable populations include the following:
  - Increasing the number of people who have a routine primary care provider
  - Increasing the number of people with health insurance
  - Reducing the number of people who are unable or have a delay in accessing health care services and prescribed medications

VIOLENCE

- Types of Violence Within Communities
  - Homicide
    - Homicide is often related to substance use.
    - Most homicides are committed by someone known to the victim and occur during an argument.
    - Abuse often precedes homicide within families.
    - Rates are increasing among adolescents.
  - Assault
    - Males are more likely to be assaulted.
    - Youths are at a significantly higher risk.

- Rape
  - Rape is often unreported.
    - It includes date and marital rape.
    - The majority of violence against women is intimate partner violence.
    - Incidence is higher in cities, between 8 p.m. and 2 a.m., on the weekends, and in the summer months.
- Suicide
  - Women report attempting suicide more often than men.
  - Rates of suicide are highest in men and individuals over the age of 65.
  - Risk factors for suicide include depression or other mental disorders, substance use, and intimate partner issues.
- Abuse
  - Physical violence occurs when pain or harm results:
    - Toward an infant or child, as is the case with shaken baby syndrome (caused by violent shaking of young infants).
    - Toward a domestic partner, such as striking or strangling the partner.
    - Toward an older adult in the home (elder abuse), such as pushing an older adult parent and causing her to fall.
  - Sexual violence occurs when sexual contact takes place without consent, whether the victim is able or unable to give that consent.
  - Emotional violence, which includes behavior that minimizes an individual's feelings of self-worth or humiliates, threatens, or intimidates a family member.
  - Neglect includes the failure to provide the following:
    - Physical care, such as food, shelter, and hygiene
    - Emotional care and/or stimulation necessary to achieve developmental milestones, such as speaking and interacting with a child
    - Education for a child
    - Needed health or dental care
  - Economic Maltreatment
    - Failure to provide the needs of a victim when adequate funds are available
    - Unpaid bills when another person is managing the finances
    - Theft of or misuse of money or property

- Individual Assessment for Violence
  - Factors influencing an individual's potential for violence
    - History of being abused or exposure to violence
    - Low self-esteem
    - Fear and distrust of others
    - Poor self-control
    - Inadequate social skills
    - Minimal social support/isolation
    - Immature motivation for marriage or childbearing
    - Weak coping skills
- Recognizing Actual or Potential Child Abuse/Neglect
  - Unexplained injury
  - Unusual fear of the nurse and others
  - Injuries/wounds not mentioned in history
  - Fractures, including older healed fractures
  - Presence of injuries/wounds/fractures in various stages of healing
  - Subdural hematomas
  - Trauma to genitalia
  - Malnourishment or dehydration
  - General poor hygiene or inappropriate dress for weather conditions
  - Considered to be a "bad child"
- Recognizing Potential or Actual Older Adult Abuse
  - Unexplained or repeated physical injuries
  - Physical neglect and unmet basic needs
  - Rejection of assistance by caregiver
  - Financial mismanagement
  - Withdrawal and passivity
  - Depression
- Community Assessment: Social and Community Factors Influencing Violence
  - Work stress
  - Unemployment
  - Media exposure to violence
  - Crowded living conditions
  - Poverty
  - Feelings of powerlessness
  - Social isolation
  - Lack of community resources (playgrounds, parks, theaters)

- Strategies to reduce societal violence

STRATEGIES TO REDUCE SOCIETAL VIOLENCE

Primary Prevention

› Teach alternative methods of conflict resolution, anger management, and coping strategies in community settings.

› Organize parenting classes to provide anticipatory guidance of expected age-appropriate behaviors, appropriate parental responses, and forms of discipline.

› Educate clients about community services that are available to provide protection from violence.

› Promote public understanding about the aging process and about safeguards to ensure a safe and secure environment for older adults in the community.

› Assist in removing or reducing factors that contribute to stress by referring caretakers of older adult clients to respite services, assisting an unemployed parent in finding employment, or increasing social support networks for socially isolated families.

› Encourage older adults and their families to safeguard their funds and property by getting more information about a financial representative trust, durable power of attorney, a representative payee, and joint tenancy.

› Teach individuals that no one has a right to touch or hurt another person, and make sure they know how to report cases of abuse.

Secondary Prevention

› Identify and screen those at risk for abuse and individuals who are potential abusers.

› Assess and evaluate any unexplained bruises or injuries of any individual.

› Screen all pregnant women for potential abuse. This may be the one time in some women's lives that they may access the health care system on a regular basis.

› Refer sexual assault or rape victims to a local emergency department for assessment by a sexual assault abuse team. Caution the client not to bathe following the assault because it will destroy physical evidence.

› Assess and counsel anyone contemplating suicide or homicide and refer the individual to the appropriate services.

› Support and educate the offender, even though a report must be made.

› Assess and help offenders address and deal with the stressors that may be causing or contributing to the abuse, such as mental illness or substance use.

› Alert all involved about available resources within the community.

› Advocate for legislation designed to assist older adult independence and caregivers and to increase funding for programs that supply services to low-income, at-risk individuals.

Tertiary Prevention

› Establish parameters for long-term follow-up and supervision.

› Make resources in the community available to the client (telephone numbers of crisis lines and shelters).

› If court systems are involved, work with parents while the child is out of the home (in foster care).

› Refer to mental health professionals for long-term assistance.

› Provide grief counseling to families of suicide or homicide victims.

› Develop support groups for caregivers and victims of violence.

Q
PCC

- When caring for clients who experience violence:
  - Build trust and confidence with a client.
  - Focus on the client rather than the situation.
  - Assess for immediate danger.
  - Provide emergency care as needed.
  - Develop a plan for safety.
  - Make needed referrals for community services and legal options.
  - If abuse has occurred, complete mandatory reporting, following agency guidelines.

SUBSTANCE USE DISORDERS

- Substance use disorders involve the maladaptive use of substances resulting in threats to an individual's health or social and economic functioning.
- Substance use and addictive disorders have significant effects on family dynamics, and often lead to codependency.
- Substance use disorders negatively affect family life, public safety, and the economy.
- Dependence is a pattern of pathological, compulsive use of substances and involves physiological and psychological dependence.
  - Cardinal signs of dependence include manifestations of tolerance and withdrawal.
  - Denial is also a primary sign of dependence and may include the following:
    - Defensiveness
    - Lying about use
    - Minimizing use
    - Blaming or rationalizing use
    - Intellectualizing
- Alcohol, tobacco, and other substance use and addictive disorders can cause multiple health problems, including the following:
  - Low birth weight
  - Congenital abnormalities
  - Accidents
  - Homicides
  - Suicides
  - Chronic diseases
  - Violence
- Recovery from substance use and addictive disorders occurs over years and usually involves relapses. A strong support system, including 12-step programs and self-help groups for family members, is important.
- Community health nurses are front-line health professionals who are able to assist those with substance use and addiction disorders.

- Alcohol Use
  - Alcohol is the most commonly used substance in the United States. It is socially acceptable, as well as easily accessible.
  - Alcohol is a depressant. Alcohol dulls the senses to outside stimulation and sedates the inhibitory centers in the brain.
  - The direct effect of alcohol is determined by the blood alcohol level.
    - The body processes alcohol dependent on several factors, including the following:
      - The size and weight of the drinker
      - Gender (affects metabolism)
      - Carbonation (increases absorption)
      - Time elapsed during alcohol consumption
      - Food in the stomach
      - The drinker's emotional state
    - The body burns about 0.5 oz of alcohol per hr.
    - Excess alcohol that is not metabolized circulates in the blood and affects the central nervous system and the brain.
  - People who frequently and consistently drink alcohol develop a tolerance, an increased requirement for alcohol to achieve the desired effect.
  - Following prolonged use, manifestations of alcohol withdrawal appears within 4 to 12 hr.
    - Manifestations of withdrawal include the following:
      - Irritability
      - Tremors
      - Nausea
      - Vomiting
      - Headaches
      - Diaphoresis
      - Anxiety
      - Sleep disturbances
      - Tachycardia
      - Elevated blood pressure
    - Increased blood pressure, tachycardia, and diaphoresis are indicators of delirium tremens or alcohol withdrawal delirium.
    - The prompt use of benzodiazepines at the onset of symptoms can prevent the serious complication of delirium tremens.
    - It is important to determine the last drink the client has taken in order to accurately assess for signs of withdrawal and delirium tremens.

- Tobacco Use

  - Smoking is the most important preventable cause of death in the United States, according to the Centers for Disease Control and Prevention.

  - Nicotine is a stimulant that temporarily creates a feeling of alertness and energy. Repeated use to avoid the subsequent "down" that will follow this period of stimulation leads to a vicious cycle of use and physical dependence (withdrawal effects if not consumed).

  - Tolerance to nicotine develops quickly.

  - Cigarette smoking results in deep inhalation of smoke, which poses the greatest health risk (cancer, cardiovascular disease, respiratory disease); however, cigars, pipes, and smokeless tobacco increase the risk of cancers of the lips, mouth, and throat. Secondhand smoke poses considerable health risks (respiratory disease, lung cancer) to nonsmokers.

- Other Drugs

  - Other stimulants include caffeine, amphetamines, methamphetamines, and cocaine.

  - Other depressants include barbiturates, benzodiazepines, chloral hydrate, and GHB.

  - Opiates include morphine, heroin, codeine, and fentanyl.

  - Hallucinogens (psychedelics) produce anxiety, paranoia, impaired judgment, and hallucinations. Some examples are lysergic acid diethylamide (LSD), phencyclidine (PCP), and MDMA (Ecstasy).

  - Inhalants are volatile substances that are inhaled ("huffed"). Death may result from acute cardiac dysrhythmias or asphyxiation.

- Individual Assessment

  - Establish rapport with the client. Pose questions in a matter-of-fact tone. Be nonjudgmental. Communicate that the purpose of questioning is because of the effects that different practices can have on an individual's health. Use the communication technique of normalizing when appropriate.

  - Seek information about specific substances used, methods of use, and the quantity (packs, ounces) and frequency of use.

  - Elicit information about consequences experienced (blackouts, overdoses, injuries to self/others, legal or social difficulties).

  - Determine if the individual perceives a substance use problem.

  - Discuss the individual's history of previous rehabilitation experiences.

  - Gather family history of substance use and social exposure to other substance users.

  - Some physical assessment findings include the following:

    - Vital signs – Varies depending on substance being used.

    - Appearance – Individual can appear disheveled with an unsteady gait.

    - Eyes – Pupils can appear dilated or pinpoint, red, also poor eye contact.

    - Skin – Can be diaphoretic, cool, and/or clammy; needle track marks or spider angiomas may be visible.

    - Nose – Can be runny, congested, red and/or cauliflower-shaped.

    - Tremors – Fine or coarse tremors may be present.

- Strategies to Reduce Substance Use Disorders

STRATEGIES TO REDUCE SUBSTANCE USE DISORDERS
Primary Prevention
› Increase public awareness, particularly among young people, regarding the hazards and addictive qualities of substance use (e.g., public education campaigns, school education programs).
› Encourage development of life skills.
Secondary Prevention
› Identify at-risk individuals and assist them to reduce sources of stress, including possible referral to social services to eliminate financial difficulties or other sources of stress.
› Screen individuals for maladaptive substance use.
Tertiary Prevention
› Assist the client to develop a plan to avoid high-risk situations and to enhance coping and lifestyle changes.
› Refer the client to community groups, such as Alcoholics Anonymous (AA) and Narcotics Anonymous (NA).
› Monitor pharmacological management.
› Provide emotional support to recovering abusers and their families, including positive reinforcement.

MENTAL HEALTH

- Mental Illness Characteristics
  - Occurs across the lifespan
  - High risk of substance use disorders
  - High suicide risk
  - Specific disorders include:
    - Affective disorders (bipolar disorder, major depression)
    - Anxiety disorders (obsessive-compulsive, panic, phobias, posttraumatic stress)
    - Schizophrenia
    - Dementia
    - Conduct disorders
    - Eating disorders
- Factors Contributing to Mental Health of Aggregates
  - Individual coping abilities
  - Stressful life events (exposure to violence)
  - Social events (recent divorce, separation, unemployment, bereavement)
  - Chronic health problems
  - Stigma associated with seeking mental health services

- Strategies for Improving Mental Health

STRATEGIES FOR IMPROVING MENTAL HEALTH
Primary Prevention
› Educate populations regarding mental health issues.
› Teach stress-reduction techniques.
› Provide parenting classes.
› Provide bereavement support.
› Promote protective factors (coping abilities) and risk factor reduction.
Secondary Prevention
› Screen to detect mental health disorders.
› Work directly with at-risk individuals, families, and groups through the formation of a therapeutic relationship.
› Conduct crisis intervention.
Tertiary Prevention
› Perform medication monitoring.
› Provide mental health interventions.
› Make referrals to various groups of professionals, including support groups.
› Maintain the client's level of function to prevent relapse or frequent rehospitalization.
› Identify behavioral, environmental, and biological triggers that may lead to relapse.
› Assist the client in planning a regular lifestyle and minimizing sources of stress.
› Educate the client and family regarding medication side effects, potential interactions.

HOMELESSNESS

- Homeless Population Characteristics
  - Adults who are unemployed, earn low wages, or are migrant workers
  - Female heads of household
  - Families with children (fastest growing segment)
  - People who have a mental illness (large segment)
  - Veterans
  - People who have substance use and addictive disorders
  - Unaccompanied youth
  - Adolescent runaways
  - Intimate partner abuse victims
  - People who have HIV or AIDS
  - Older adults with no place to go and no support system
- Health Issues of Homeless Populations
  - Upper respiratory disorders
  - Tuberculosis

- ○ Skin disorders (athlete's foot) and infestations (scabies, lice)
- ○ Substance use disorders
- ○ HIV/AIDS
- ○ Trauma
- ○ Mental illness
- ○ Dental caries
- ○ Hypothermia and heat-related illnesses
- ○ Malnutrition
- Strategies for Preventing Homelessness and Assisting Individuals Who are Homeless
  - ○ Prevent individuals and families from becoming homeless by assisting them in eliminating factors that may contribute to homelessness.
    - ▪ Refer those with underlying mental health disorders to therapy and counseling.
    - ▪ Enhance parenting skills that may prevent young people from feeling the need to run away.
  - ○ Alleviate existing homelessness by making referrals for financial assistance, food supplements, and health services.
    - ▪ Assist homeless clients in locating temporary shelter.
    - ▪ Assist clients in finding ways to meet long-term shelter needs.
    - ▪ If homeless shelters are not provided in the community, work with government officials to develop shelter programs.
  - ○ Prevent recurrence of poverty, homelessness, and health problems that result in conditions of poverty and homelessness.
    - ▪ Advocate and provide efforts toward political activity to provide needed services for people who have a mental illness and are homeless.
    - ▪ Make referrals for employee assistance and educational programs to allow clients who are homeless to eliminate the factors contributing to their homelessness.

RURAL AND MIGRANT HEALTH

- Health Status of Rural Residents
  - ○ Higher infant and maternal morbidity rates
  - ○ Higher rates of diabetes mellitus
  - ○ More likely to be obese
  - ○ Less likely to meet physical activity recommendations
  - ○ Higher rates of suicide
  - ○ Increased trauma/injuries from lightning, farm machinery, drowning, and boating, snowmobile, all-terrain vehicle, and motorcycle crashes
  - ○ Increased occupational-associated risks (agriculture, fishing, mining, and construction are the most dangerous industries)
  - ○ Less likely to seek preventive care
- Barriers to Health Care in Rural Areas
  - ○ Distance from services

- ○ Lack of personal/public transportation
- ○ Unpredictable weather and/or travel conditions
- ○ Inability to pay for care/underinsured/uninsured
- ○ Shortage of rural hospitals/health care providers
- Health Problems of Migrant Workers
  - ○ Dental disease
  - ○ Tuberculosis
  - ○ Chronic conditions
  - ○ Stress, anxiety, and other mental health concerns
  - ○ Leukemia
  - ○ Iron deficiency anemia
  - ○ Stomach, uterine, and cervical cancers
  - ○ Lack of prenatal care
  - ○ Higher infant mortality rates
- Issues in Migrant Health
  - ○ Poor and unsanitary working and housing conditions
  - ○ Exposure to environmental pesticides
  - ○ Less access to dental, mental health, and pharmacy services
  - ○ Inability to afford care
  - ○ Availability of services (distance, transportation, hours of service, health record tracking)
  - ○ Language barriers and cultural aspects of health care
- Strategies for Rural and Migrant Health Care

STRATEGIES FOR RURAL AND MIGRANT HEALTH CARE
Primary Prevention
› Educate regarding measures to reduce exposure to pesticides.
› Teach regarding accident prevention measures.
› Provide prenatal care.
› Mobilize preventive services (dental, immunizations).
Secondary Prevention
› Screen for pesticide exposure.
› Screen for skin cancer.
› Screen for chronic preventable diseases.
› Screen for communicable diseases.
Tertiary Prevention
› Treat for symptoms of pesticide exposure.
› Mobilize primary care and emergency services.

VETERANS

- There are approximately 25 million veterans in the United States.
  - Approximately 2 million are women.
  - Approximately 9 million are over the age of 65.
- Veterans Health Administration (within the U.S. Department of Veterans Affairs) is responsible for purchasing coverage and delivering health care to veterans and dependents.
  - Nation's largest integrated health care system
  - Inpatient and outpatient services include the following:
    - Hospitals
    - Outpatient clinics
    - Home health services
    - Hospice and palliative care services
    - Nursing homes
    - Residential rehabilitation treatment programs
    - Readjustment counseling centers
- Veterans Health Issues
  - Mental health conditions (posttraumatic stress disorder, traumatic stress reactions, anger, depression)
  - Substance use and addiction disorders
  - Suicide
  - Infectious diseases
  - Exposures to herbicides, chemicals, and radiation
  - Traumatic brain injuries
  - Spinal cord injuries
  - Traumatic amputations
  - Cold injury
  - Military sexual trauma
  - Hearing impairments
  - Visual impairments
- Strategies for Veteran Health Care
  - Coordinate referrals to available veteran resources.
  - Advocate for continued strengthening of the Veterans Health Administration health care system.
  - Assist clients to transition from active duty status to veteran.
  - Ensure continuity of care between hospital and outpatient settings.

○ Develop partnerships with local agencies to strengthen resources and achieve mutual goals.

  ▪ Possible stakeholders for partnerships

    □ State and local veteran groups

    □ Offices of rural health

    □ Local aging services

    □ Community service organizations

    □ State and local health departments

    □ Faith-based organizations

    □ Public safety departments

    □ Various media outlets

    □ Employment services

APPLICATION EXERCISES

1. A nurse at a community clinic is conducting a well-child visit with a preschool-age child. The nurse should identify which of the following as a manifestation of child neglect? (Select all that apply.)

_____ A. Underweight

_____ B. Healing spiral fracture of the arm

_____ C. Genital irritation

_____ D. Burns on the palms of the hands

_____ E. Poor hygiene

2. A nurse is caring for a client who is experiencing alcohol withdrawal. Which of the following findings is a manifestation of withdrawal?

A. Decreased blood pressure

B. Diaphoresis

C. Pin-point pupils

D. Bradycardia

3. A community health nurse is developing an education program on substance use disorders for a group of adolescents. Which of the following should the nurse include when discussing nicotine and smoking?

A. Smoking is the fifth-most preventable cause of death in the United States.

B. Nicotine is a central nervous system depressant.

C. Withdrawal effects from smoking are minimal.

D. Tolerance to nicotine develops quickly.

4. A community health nurse is developing strategies to prevent or improve mental health issues in the local area. In which of the following situations is the nurse implementing a tertiary prevention strategy?

A. Providing support programs for new parents

B. Screening a client whose spouse recently died for suicide risk

C. Teaching a client who has schizophrenia about medication interactions

D. Discussing stress reduction techniques with employees at an industrial site

5. A nurse at an urban community health agency is developing an education program for city leaders about homelessness. Which of the following should the nurse include as the fastest-growing segment of the homeless population?

    A. Families with children

    B. Adolescent runaways

    C. Intimate partner abuse victims

    D. Older adults

6. A nurse is reviewing data that will assist with the development of a program to improve health outcomes of vulnerable populations. Use the ATI Active Learning Template: Basic Concept to complete this item to include the following:

    A. Related Content: At least two national health goals that address vulnerable populations

    B. Underlying Principles: At least three issues that affect vulnerable populations

    C. Nursing Interventions: At least two strategies to improve access to health care for vulnerable populations

APPLICATION EXERCISES KEY

1. A. **CORRECT:** An underweight child is a manifestation of child neglect.

    B. INCORRECT: A healing spiral fracture is a manifestation of physical abuse.

    C. INCORRECT: Genital irritation is a manifestation of sexual abuse.

    D. INCORRECT: Burns on the palms of the hands are a manifestation of physical abuse.

    E. **CORRECT:** Poor hygiene is manifestation of child neglect.

    Ⓝ NCLEX® Connection: Psychosocial Integrity, Abuse/Neglect

2. A. INCORRECT: Increased, not decreased, blood pressure is a manifestation of alcohol withdrawal.

    B. **CORRECT:** Diaphoresis is a manifestation of alcohol withdrawal.

    C. INCORRECT: Dilated, not pin-point, pupils are a manifestation of alcohol withdrawal.

    D. INCORRECT: Tachycardia, not bradycardia, is a manifestation of alcohol withdrawal.

    Ⓝ NCLEX® Connection: Reduction of Risk Potential, System Specific Assessments

3. A. INCORRECT: Smoking is the first-most, not fifth-most, preventable cause of death in the United States.

    B. INCORRECT: Nicotine is a central nervous system stimulant, not depressant.

    C. INCORRECT: Withdrawal effects from smoking are substantial, not minimal, and increase physical dependence.

    D. **CORRECT:** Tolerance to nicotine does develop quickly.

    Ⓝ NCLEX® Connection: Health Promotion and Maintenance, Health Promotion/Disease Prevention

4. A. INCORRECT: Providing support programs for new parents is a primary prevention strategy.

    B. INCORRECT: Screening a client whose spouse recently died for suicide risk is a secondary prevention strategy.

    C. **CORRECT:** Teaching a client who has schizophrenia about medication interactions is a tertiary prevention strategy.

    D. INCORRECT: Discussing stress reduction techniques with employees at an industrial site is a primary prevention strategy.

    Ⓝ NCLEX® Connection: Health Promotion and Maintenance, High Risk Behaviors

5. A. **CORRECT:** Families with children are the fasting-growing segment of the homeless population.

    B. INCORRECT: Adolescent runaways are not the fastest-growing segment of the homeless population.

    C. INCORRECT: Intimate partner abuse victims are not the fastest-growing segment of the homeless population.

    D. INCORRECT: Older adults are not the fastest-growing segment of the homeless population.

    (N) NCLEX® Connection: Health Promotion and Maintenance, Health Promotion/Disease Prevention

6. *Using the ATI Active Learning Template: Basic Concept*

    A. Related Content
    - Increase the number of people who have a routine primary care provider.
    - Increase the number of people who have health insurance.
    - Reduce the number of people who are unable or have a delay in accessing health care services and prescribed medications.

    B. Underlying Principles
    - Violence
    - Substance use disorders
    - Homelessness
    - Mental health issues
    - Poverty
    - Chronic stress
    - Poor self-esteem
    - Access to health care services

    C. Nursing Interventions
    - Coordinate services at a central location.
    - Develop programs that goes to the population to deliver health care (home visits, health services bus, on-site clinics).
    - Create partnerships to provide free or reduced health care services.
    - Advocate for increased availability of health insurance for the uninsured and underinsured.
    - Evaluate current health care systems and make recommendations that will strengthen access.
    - Collaborate with community leaders to improve/increase the availability of public transportation.
    - Ensure the availability of translators with medical training.

    (N) NCLEX® Connection: Health Promotion and Maintenance, Health Promotion/Disease Prevention

CHAPTER 6   Communicable Diseases, Disasters, and Bioterrorism

NCLEX® CONNECTIONS

When reviewing the chapters in this unit, keep in mind the relevant sections of the NCLEX® outline, in particular:

Client Needs: Safety and Infection Control

› Relevant topics/tasks include:

» Emergency Response Plan

› Use clinical decision-making/critical thinking for emergency response plan.

» Handling Hazardous and Infectious Materials

› Identify biohazardous, flammable and infectious materials.

» Standard Precautions/Transmission-Based Precautions/Surgical Asepsis

› Understand communicable diseases and the modes of organism transmission.

Client Needs: Health Promotion and Maintenance

› Relevant topics/tasks include:

» Health Promotion/Disease Prevention

› Identify risk factors for disease/illness.

› Provide information about health promotion and maintenance recommendations (e.g., physician visits, immunizations).

chapter 6

Overview

- Large-scale events have highlighted the need for health care professionals to have knowledge of communicable disease, disaster management, and bioterrorism.
- Communicable disease is an international health concern.
- Nurses have unique skills required to plan for and respond to natural and man-made disasters.

Communicable Diseases

- Worldwide, communicable diseases are responsible for the deaths of millions each year.
- Leading causes of communicable disease deaths include acute respiratory infections (including pneumonia and influenza), AIDS, diarrheal diseases, tuberculosis, malaria, and measles.
- Populations at risk for communicable disease include the following:
  - Young children
  - Older adults
  - Immunosuppressed clients
  - Clients who have a high-risk lifestyle
  - International travelers
  - Health care workers
- The Centers for Disease Control and Prevention (CDC) recommend routine immunizations according to age. Recommendations include schedules/guidelines for children, adolescents, and adults. A "catch up" schedule and recommendations for health care personnel are also available. The CDC website (www.cdc.gov) provides a high-quality resource for the most current information regarding immunization guidelines.
- Modes of Transmission
  - Airborne (inhaled by a susceptible host)
    - Measles
    - Chickenpox
    - Tuberculosis (pulmonary or laryngeal)
    - Pertussis
    - Influenza
  - Foodborne
    - Food infection (bacterial, viral, parasitic infection of food)
      - Salmonellosis
      - Hepatitis A
      - Trichinosis
      - *Escherichia coli* (*E. coli*)

- Food intoxication (toxins produced through bacterial growth, chemical contamination, or disease-producing substances)
  - *Staphylococcus aureus*
  - *Clostridium botulinum*
- Waterborne (fecal contamination of water)
  - Cholera
  - Typhoid fever
  - Bacillary dysentery
  - *Giardia lamblia*
- Vector-borne (via a carrier such as a mosquito or tick)
  - Lyme disease
  - Rocky Mountain spotted fever
  - Malaria
- Direct contact (transmission of infectious agent from infected host to susceptible host via direct contact)
  - Sexually transmitted infections (HIV, gonorrhea, syphilis, genital herpes, hepatitis B, C, D)
  - Infectious mononucleosis
  - Enterobiasis (pinworms)
  - Impetigo, lice, scabies
- Portals of Entry and Exit
  - Portals of entry
    - Respiratory passages
    - Gastrointestinal tract
    - Skin
    - Mucous membranes
    - Genitourinary tract
    - Eyes
    - Blood vessels
  - Portals of exit
    - Respiratory secretions
    - Feces
    - Blood
    - Semen
    - Vaginal secretions
    - Saliva
    - Skin lesion exudates

- Defense Mechanisms

  ○ Herd immunity (protection due to the immunity of most community members making exposure unlikely)

  ○ Natural immunity (natural defense mechanisms of the body to resist specific antigens or toxins)

  ○ Acquired immunity (develops through actual exposure to the infectious agent)

    ▪ Active (production of antibodies by the body in response to infection or immunization with a specific antigen)

    ▪ Passive (transfer of antibodies to the host either transplacentally from mother to newborn, or through transfusions of immunoglobulins, plasma proteins, or antitoxins)

- Prevention and Control of Communicable Diseases

  ○ Communicable disease surveillance

    ▪ The community health nurse engages in communicable disease surveillance, which includes the systematic collection and analysis of data regarding infectious diseases.

    ▪ Reporting of communicable diseases is mandated by state and local regulations, and state notification to the CDC is voluntary. Nationally Notifiable Diseases include the following:

      □ Anthrax

      □ Botulism

      □ Cholera

      □ Diphtheria

      □ Giardiasis

      □ Gonorrhea

      □ Hepatitis A-C

      □ HIV infection

      □ Influenza-associated pediatric mortality

      □ Legionellosis/Legionnaires' disease

      □ Lyme disease

      □ Malaria

      □ Meningococcal disease

      □ Mumps

      □ Pertussis

      □ Poliomyelitis, paralytic

      □ Poliovirus infection, nonparalytic

      □ Rabies (human or animal)

      □ Rubella (German measles)

      □ Rubella, congenital syndrome

      □ Salmonellosis

- Severe acute respiratory syndrome-associated coronavirus disease (SARS-CoV)
- Shigellosis
- Smallpox
- Syphilis
- Tetanus
- Toxic shock syndrome
- Tuberculosis
- Typhoid fever
- Vancomycin-resistant *Staphylococcus aureus* (VRSA)

○ Health care goals regarding the control of communicable diseases

- Reductions in:
  - Infections caused by pathogens often transmitted through food
  - New HIV diagnoses among adolescents and adults
  - New AIDS cases among adolescents and adults
  - Number of perinatally acquired HIV and AIDS cases
  - Deaths from HIV infection
  - Vaccine-preventable diseases (reductions in or elimination of)
  - Number of antibiotic courses for ear infections in young children

- Increases in:
  - Consumers who follow food safety practices
  - Surviving more than 3 years after a diagnosis with AIDS
  - Adolescents and adults who have been tested for HIV in the past 12 months
  - Adults with tuberculosis (TB) who have been tested for HIV
  - Substance abuse treatment facilities that offer HIV/AIDS education, counseling, and support
  - Sexually active persons who use condoms
  - Immunization rates among young children
  - Immunization rates among adolescents
  - Annual seasonal influenza immunizations among children and adults
  - Adults who are immunized against pneumococcal disease
  - Adults who are immunized against zoster (shingles)
  - Tuberculosis clients who complete therapy

- Immunization
  - The community health nurse plays a major role in increasing immunization coverage.
  - Immunizations are often administered in community health settings, such as public health departments.
  - The community health nurse often tracks immunization schedules of at-risk populations such as children, older adults, immunosuppressed individuals, and health care workers.
  - The community health nurse must educate the community about the importance of immunizations.
  - The community health nurse must stay up to date on current immunization schedule recommendations and appropriate precautions when administering immunizations.
- Levels of prevention

LEVELS OF PREVENTION OF COMMUNICABLE DISEASES
Primary Prevention
› Prevent the occurrence of infectious disease.
› Educate the public regarding the need for immunizations, and federal and state vaccination programs.
› Counsel clients traveling to other countries about protection from infectious diseases. Refer clients to the health department for information about mandatory immunizations.
› Educate the public regarding prevention of disease and ways to eliminate risk factors for exposure, such as hand hygiene, universal precautions, proper food handling and storage, and use of condoms.
Secondary Prevention
› Increase early detection through screening and case finding.
› Refer suspected cases of communicable disease for diagnostic confirmation and epidemiologic reporting.
› Provide postexposure prophylaxis (hepatitis A, rabies).
› Quarantine clients when necessary.
Tertiary Prevention
› Decrease complications and disabilities due to infectious diseases through treatment and rehabilitation.
› Monitor treatment compliance, including directly observed therapy.
› Identify and link clients to needed community resources.

Disasters

- A disaster is an event that causes human suffering and demands more resources than are available in the community. A disaster may be man-made, naturally occurring, or a combination of both, such as a natural disaster causing technological failures.
- Four Levels of Disaster Management
  - Disaster prevention
    - Includes activities to prevent natural and man-made disasters, such as increasing surveillance, improving inspections and airport security, and strengthening public health processes such as immunizations, isolation, and quarantine.
    - Activities such as strengthening levies/barriers to prevent flooding and teaching methods of preventing communicable disease transmission are also a component of disaster prevention.

- The community's threats, vulnerabilities, and capabilities are determined as part of disaster prevention, as are the demographics of community members.

- This level also includes identification and assessment of populations at risk.

  □ Populations at risk are those populations that have fewer resources or less of an ability to withstand and survive a disaster without physical harm.

  □ These populations tend to be physically isolated, disabled, or unable to access disaster services. Strategic emergency planning is necessary to prevent the loss of lives in susceptible populations.

○ Disaster preparedness

- Disaster preparedness occurs at the national, state, and local levels. Personal and family preparedness are crucial components of disaster preparedness, as is professional preparedness for individuals employed in civil service and health care.

- Disaster preparations should stem from threats and vulnerabilities identified in the prevention level, and should coordinate community efforts as well as outline specific roles of local agencies.

- This level of management includes preparedness for natural or man-made disasters.

- Individual and family disaster preparedness include creating an action plan and determining alternative methods of communication, highlighting possible evacuation routes, identifying local and distant meeting places, and creating a disaster kit.

- Setting up a communication protocol is an important part of community disaster planning. The communication plan should provide for access to emergency agencies, such as the American Red Cross, and state and federal government agencies.

- Disaster drills mock possible scenarios in the local area and enhance preparedness of community members, government agencies, health care facilities, and businesses.

○ Disaster response

- Different agencies, governmental and nongovernmental, are responsible for different levels of disaster response. Some of the agencies with a role in disaster response include the Federal Emergency Management Agency (FEMA), the CDC, U.S. Department of Homeland Security (DHS), American Red Cross, Office of Emergency Management (OEM), and the public health system.

- Disaster management response includes an initial assessment of the span of the disaster.

  □ How many people are affected?

  □ How many are injured or dead?

  □ How much fresh water and food is available?

  □ What are the areas of risk or sanitation problems?

- Disasters are classified according to type, level, and scope.

- If a federal emergency is declared, the National Response Framework (NRF) is activated and provides direction for an organized, effective national response.

- Disaster recovery

  - Recovery begins when danger no longer exists and needed representatives and agencies are available to assist with rebuilding.

  - Recovery lasts until the economic and civil life of the community are restored, which can be days, weeks, or even years. At an individual level, it is the time it takes an individual to become functional within a community after a disaster.

  - Communicable disease and sanitation controls are important aspects of disaster recovery.

  - Posttraumatic stress disorder (PTSD) and delayed stress reactions (DSR) are common during the aftermath of disasters and may affect both caregivers and victims.

  - Phases of emotional reaction during a disaster

    - Heroic – Intense excitement and concern for survival. Often a rush of assistance from outside the area is present.

    - Honeymoon – Affected individuals begin to bond and relive their experiences.

    - Disillusionment – Responders may experience depression and exhaustion. Phase contains unexpected delays in receiving aid.

    - Reconstruction – Involves adjusting to a new reality and continued rebuilding of the area. Counseling is sometimes needed. Those affected begin looking ahead.

- Roles of Community Health Nurses in Disaster Management

  - Participation in risk assessment includes asking the following questions:

    - What are the populations at risk within the community?

    - Have there been previous disasters, natural or man-made?

    - What size of an area or population is likely to be affected in a worst-case scenario?

    - What is the community disaster plan?

    - What kind of warning system is in place?

    - What types of disaster response teams (volunteers, nurses, health professionals, emergency medical technicians, firemen) are in place?

    - What kinds of resource facilities (hospitals, shelters, churches, food-storage facilities) are available in the event of a disaster?

    - What type of evacuation measures (boat, motor vehicle, train) will be needed?

    - What type of environmental dangers (chemical plants, sewage displacement) may be involved?

  - Participation in disaster planning includes the following:

    - Developing a disaster response plan based on the most probable disaster threats.

    - Identifying the community disaster warning system and communication center, and learning how to access it.

    - Identifying the first responders in the community disaster plan.

    - Making a list of agencies that are available for the varying levels of disaster management at the local, state, and national levels.

    - Defining the nursing roles in first priority, second priority, and third priority triage.

- Identifying the specific roles of personnel involved in disaster response and the chain of command.

- Locating all equipment and supplies needed for disaster management, including hazmat suits, infectious control items, medical supplies, food, and potable water.

  □ Detailing a plan to replenish these regularly.

- Checking equipment (including evacuation vehicles) regularly to ensure proper operation.

- Evaluating the efficiency, response time, and safety of disaster drills, mass casualty drills, and disaster plans.

○ Participation in disaster response includes the following:

- Activating the disaster management plan.

- Performing triage and directing those affected, coordinating evacuation, quarantine, and opening of shelters.

- Triaging involves identifying those who have serious versus minor injuries, prioritizing care of victims, and transferring those requiring immediate attention to medical facilities.

○ Participation in disaster recovery includes the following:

- Making home visits and reassessing the health care needs of the affected population.

- Providing and coordinating care in shelters.

- Providing stress counseling and assessing for PTSD or delayed stress reactions, and making referrals for psychological treatment.

○ Participation in evaluation of disaster response includes the following:

- Evaluating the area, effect, and level of the disaster.

- Creating ongoing assessment and surveillance reports.

- Evaluating the efficiency of the disaster response teams.

- Estimating the length of time for recovery of community services, such as electricity and running potable water.

Bioterrorism

- Agents of Bioterrorism

  ○ Category A biological agents are the highest priority agents, posing a risk to national security because they are easily transmitted and have high mortality rates.

    - Examples include smallpox (variola), botulism toxin, anthrax, tularemia, hemorrhagic viral fevers, and plague.

  ○ Category B biological agents are the second-highest priority because they are moderately easy to disseminate and have high morbidity rates and low mortality rates.

    - Examples include typhus and cholera.

  ○ Category C biological agents are the third-highest priority, comprising emerging pathogens that can be engineered for mass dissemination because they are easy to produce, and/or have a potential for high morbidity and mortality rates.

    - Examples include hantavirus.

BIOTERRORISM INCIDENTS		
INCIDENT	**MANIFESTATIONS**	**TREATMENT/PREVENTION**
Inhalational anthrax	› Headache › Fever › Muscle aches › Chest discomfort › Severe dyspnea › Shock	› IV ciprofloxacin (Cipro) prophylactically for exposure or high risk of exposure › Antibiotics do not stop disease progression.
Botulism	› Difficulty swallowing › Progressive weakness › Nausea, vomiting, abdominal cramps › Difficulty breathing	› Airway management › Antitoxin › Elimination of toxin › Supportive care – nutrition, fluids, prevent complications
Smallpox	› High fever › Fatigue › Severe headache › Rash (begins on face and tongue, quickly spreading to the trunk, arms, and legs, then hands and feet) that turns to pus-filled lesions › Vomiting	› Treatment – no cure › Supportive care – hydration, pain medication, antipyretics › Prevention – vaccine (provides 10 years of immunity)
Ebola	› Fever › Hemorrhage › Vomiting, diarrhea › Cough › Jaundice › Shock	› Treatment – no cure › Airway management › Dialysis › Supportive care – psychological support for client and family › Prevention – avoidance of contaminated items/animals

- Delivery Mechanisms for Biological Agents
    - Direct contact (subcutaneous anthrax)
    - Simple dispersal device (airborne, nuclear)
    - Water and food contamination
    - Droplet or blood contact
- Role of the Community Health Nurse
    - Participate in planning and preparation for immediate response to a bioterrorist event.
    - Identify potential biological agents for bioterrorism.
    - Survey for and report bioterrorism activity (usually to the local health department).
    - Promptly participate in measures to contain and control the spread of infections resulting from bioterrorist activity.

- Assessment of Bioterrorism Threat
  - Is the population at risk for sudden high disease rates?
  - Is the vector that normally carries a specific disease available in the geographical area affected?
  - Is there a potential delivery system within the community?
- Recognition of a Bioterrorism Event
  - Is there a rapidly increasing disease incidence in a normally healthy population?
  - Is a disease occurring that is unusual for the area?
  - Is an endemic occurring at an unusual time? For example, is there an outbreak of influenza in the summer?
  - Are there large numbers of people dying rapidly with similar presenting symptoms?
  - Are there any individuals presenting with unusual symptoms?
  - Are there unusual numbers of dead or dying animals, unusual liquids/vapors/odors?

BIOTERRORISM LEVELS OF PREVENTION

Primary Prevention

› Preparation with bioterrorism drills, vaccines, and ensuring availability of antibiotics for exposure prophylaxis
› Bioterrorism planning
   » Design a bioterrorist response plan using the most probable biological agent in the local area.
   » Identify the chain of command for reporting bioterrorist attacks.
   » Define the nursing roles in the event of a bioterrorist attack.
   » Set up protocols for different levels of infection control and containment.

Secondary Prevention

› Early recognition
› Activation of bioterrorism response plan in response to a bioterrorist event
› Immediate implementation of infection control and containment measures, including decontamination, environmental disinfection, protective equipment, community education/notification, and quarantines
› Screening the population for exposure, assessing rates of infection, and administering vaccines as available
› Assisting with and educating the population regarding symptom identification and management (immunoglobulin, antiviral, antitoxins, and antibiotic therapy, depending on the agent)
› Monitoring mortality and morbidity

Tertiary Prevention

› Rehabilitation of survivors
› Monitoring medication regimens and referrals
› Evaluating the effectiveness and timeliness of the bioterrorism plan

APPLICATION EXERCISES

1. A nurse is preparing a community health program on communicable diseases. When discussing modes of transmission, the nurse should include which of the following as an airborne illness?

    A. Cholera

    B. Malaria

    C. Influenza

    D. Salmonellosis

2. A home health nurse is discussing portals of entry with a group of newly hired assistive personnel. Which of the following are portals of entry the nurse should discuss? (Select all that apply.)

_____ A. Respiratory secretions

_____ B. Skin

_____ C. Genitourinary tract

_____ D. Saliva

_____ E. Mucous membranes

3. A newly hired public health nurse is familiarizing himself with the levels of disaster management. Which of the following actions is a component of disaster prevention?

    A. Outlining specific roles of community agencies

    B. Identifying community vulnerabilities

    C. Prioritizing care of individuals

    D. Providing stress counseling

4. A community health nurse is educating the public on the agents of bioterrorism. Which of the following are Category A biological agents? (Select all that apply.)

_____ A. Hantavirus

_____ B. Typhus

_____ C. Plague

_____ D. Tularemia

_____ E. Botulism

5. A community health nurse is determining available and needed supplies in the event of a bioterrorism attack. The nurse should be aware that community members exposed to anthrax will need access to which of the following medications?

    A. Metronidazole (Flagyl)

    B. Ciprofloxacin (Cipro)

    C. Zanamivir (Relenza)

    D. Fluconazole (Diflucan)

6. A community health nurse is responding to a man-made disaster in the local community. Using the ATI Active Learning Template: Basic Concept, complete this item to include the following:

    A. Underlying Principles:
- Three agencies involved in disaster response
- Two questions to ask to determine the disaster's scope

    B. Nursing Interventions: Four disaster response nursing roles

APPLICATION EXERCISES KEY

1. A. INCORRECT: Cholera is waterborne illness.

    B. INCORRECT: Malaria is a vector-borne illness.

    C. **CORRECT:** When discussing modes transmission, the nurse should include influenza as an airborne illness.

    D. INCORRECT: Salmonellosis is a foodborne illness.

    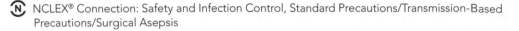 NCLEX® Connection: Safety and Infection Control, Standard Precautions/Transmission-Based Precautions/Surgical Asepsis

2. A. INCORRECT: Respiratory secretions are a portal of exit.

    B. **CORRECT:** Skin is a portal of entry the nurse should discuss.

    C. **CORRECT:** The genitourinary tract is a portal of entry the nurse should discuss.

    D. INCORRECT: Saliva is a portal of exit.

    E. **CORRECT:** Mucous membranes are a portal of entry the nurse should discuss.

    Ⓝ NCLEX® Connection: Safety and Infection Control, Standard Precautions/Transmission-Based Precautions/Surgical Asepsis

3. A. INCORRECT: Outlining specific roles of community agencies is a component of disaster preparedness.

    B. **CORRECT:** Identifying community vulnerabilities is a component of disaster prevention.

    C. INCORRECT: Prioritizing care of individuals is a component of disaster response.

    D. INCORRECT: Providing stress counseling is a component of disaster recovery.

    Ⓝ NCLEX® Connection: Safety and Infection Control, Emergency Response Plan

4. A. INCORRECT: Hantavirus is a Category C biological agent.

    B. INCORRECT: Typhus is a Category B biological agent.

    C. **CORRECT:** Plague is a Category A biological agent.

    D. **CORRECT:** Tularemia is a Category A biological agent.

    E. **CORRECT:** Botulism is a Category A biological agent.

    Ⓝ NCLEX® Connection: Safety and Infection Control, Emergency Response Plan

5.   A. INCORRECT: Metronidazole is used to treat trichomoniasis, skin infections, and septicemia.

    B. **CORRECT:** Community members exposed to anthrax will need access to ciprofloxacin. This medication is used for the prophylactic treatment of anthrax.

    C. INCORRECT: Zanamivir is used to treat influenza.

    D. INCORRECT: Fluconazole is used to treat candidiasis.

    Ⓝ NCLEX® Connection: Pharmacological and Parenteral Therapies, Medication Administration

6.   *Using the ATI Active Learning Template: Basic Concept*

    A. Underlying Principles
- Involved agencies
  - FEMA
  - CDC
  - U.S. Department of Homeland Security (DHS)
  - American Red Cross
  - Office of Emergency Management (OEM)
- Disaster scope
  - How many people are affected?
  - How many are injured or dead?
  - How much fresh water and food is available?
  - What are the areas of risk or sanitation problems?

    B. Nursing Interventions
- Nursing roles
  - Activating the disaster management plan
  - Performing triage and directing disaster victims
  - Identifying people with serious versus minor injuries
  - Prioritizing care of those affected
  - Transferring those requiring immediate attention to medical facilities
  - Coordinating evacuation or quarantines
  - Opening shelters

    Ⓝ NCLEX® Connection: Safety and Infection Control, Emergency Response Plan

CHAPTER 7   Continuity of Care

Client Needs: Management of Care

› Relevant topics/tasks include:

» Case Management

› Explore resources available to assist the client in achieving or maintaining independence.

» Collaboration with Interdisciplinary Team

› Identify significant information to report to other disciplines.

» Concepts of Management

› Act as a liaison between the client and others.

» Referrals

› Identify community resources for the client.

Overview

- Community health nurses play a large role in maintaining continuity of care for clients as they transition from inpatient to outpatient settings.

- Community health nurses use technology to maintain continuity of care.

- Community partnerships are essential to improving and maintaining healthy communities.

- Partnerships may be developed among individuals, families, community agencies, and/or citizen groups.

EXAMPLES OF PARTNERING ENTITIES		
› Individuals	› Civic organizations	› Political offices
› Families	› Citizen groups	› Employment bureaus
› Community agencies	› Educational settings	
CHARACTERISTICS OF SUCCESSFUL PARTNERSHIPS		
› Shared power	› Integrity	› Negotiation
› Shared goals	› Flexibility	

- Community health nurses should facilitate the development of partnerships within the community. These partnerships are important in the attainment of jointly desired health outcomes.

- Groups partnering to elicit needed change in the community are more powerful than a nurse working independently with an individual.

REFERRALS, DISCHARGE PLANNING, AND CASE MANAGEMENT

Overview

- A continuum of care assists in coordinating and providing individualized health care services, without disruption.

- Community health nurses facilitate continuity of care through case management services. These services include focused supervision for individualized care, follow-up, and referrals to appropriate resources.

- The establishment of an ongoing relationship between an individual and a health care provider leads to improved health outcomes.

Consultations

- A consultant is someone with specialized knowledge who provides expert advice, services, or information.

- Nursing actions related to consultations include the following:

  ○ Initiate the necessary consults or notify the provider of the client's needs so the provider can initiate a consult.

  ○ Seek expertise from health care professionals representing a variety of disciplines.

  ○ Request expert opinions of key community members, agency leaders, and other professionals.

  ○ Seek expertise of other nurses, specialty nurses (psychiatric nurse, school nurse, gerontological nurse, diabetes management nurse), or advanced practice nurses (psychiatric mental health nurse practitioner, adult nurse practitioner).

  ○ Incorporate recommendations from a consultant into the client's plan of care or program planning for the community.

  ○ Coordinate recommendations from multiple consultants (e.g., providers, advanced practice nurses, pharmacists, holistic providers) to ensure client safety.

  ○ Serve as expert witnesses in legal proceedings.

  ○ Serve as a consultant regarding the health care needs of individuals, families, and groups within the community served.

Referrals

- Referrals for individuals in acute care settings typically are based on the medical diagnosis, or other relevant clinical information. Resources assist in restoring, maintaining, or promoting health.

- The nurse assists in linking the client with community resources, and must have knowledge of individuals and organizations that can serve as resources.

- The nurse educates clients about community resources and self-care measures.

HEALTH CARE SERVICES		
› Physicians	› Long-term facilities	› Occupational therapy services
› Acute-care settings	› Home care services	› Specialty service agencies
› Primary care sites	› Rehabilitation services	› Pharmacies
› Health departments	› Physical therapy services	
SUPPORT SERVICES		
› Psychological services	› Life care planners	› Meal delivery services
› Churches	› Medical equipment providers	› Transportation services
› Support groups		

- Steps in the referral process include:
  - Engaging in a working relationship with the client.
  - Establishing criteria for the referral.
  - Exploring resources.
  - Accepting the client's decision to use a given resource.
  - Making the referral.
  - Facilitating the referral.
  - Evaluating the outcome.
- Barriers to the referral process

CLIENT BARRIERS	
› Lack of motivation	› Priorities
› Inadequate information about community resources	› Finances
› Inadequate understanding of the need for referral	› Cultural factors
› Accessibility needs	
RESOURCE BARRIERS	
› Attitudes of health care personnel	› Time limitations
› Costs of services	› Limited expertise working with culturally diverse populations
› Physical accessibility of resources	

- Follow up considerations include:
  - Monitoring to determine if the referral was completed.
  - Assessing whether referral outcomes were met.
  - Determining if the client was satisfied with the referral.

Discharge Planning

- Discharge planning is an essential component of the continuum of care, and is an ongoing assessment that anticipates the future needs of the client.
- Discharge planning requires ongoing communication between the client, nurse, providers, family, and other health care providers. The goal of discharge planning is to enhance the well-being of the client by establishing appropriate options for meeting the health care needs of the client.
- Discharge planning begins at admission.

Case Management

- Case management nursing includes the following:
  - Promoting interprofessional services and increased client/family involvement.
  - Decreasing cost by improving client outcomes.
  - Providing education to optimize health participation.
  - Advocating for services and client rights.

- Collaboration between clients, family, community resources, payer sources, and other health care professionals contributes to successful management of the client's health care needs.

- Case management nurses must possess excellent communication skills in order to facilitate communication among all parties involved. Being able to articulate the needs of the client to various parties can save time and unnecessary distress.

- Using the nursing process during case management also will help the client to obtain important services and to treat his condition.

APPLYING THE NURSING PROCESS DURING CASE MANAGEMENT	
Assessment	› Clarify the problem by evaluating physical needs, psychosocial issues, functional ability, and financial constraints.
Diagnosis	› Determine the cause and precipitating factors. › Identify applicable nursing diagnoses by using the above assessment.
Planning	› In conjunction with the interprofessional team, determine the following: » Prioritization of identified problems » Possible outcomes for the client » Advantages and disadvantages of possible outcomes » What role each participant will play » Impact on the client in each of the areas listed for the assessment
Implementation	› Contact service providers › Provide referral information › Coordinate all services to be provided
Evaluation (continued monitoring)	› Monitor the client to determine whether services are still appropriate › Monitor the care provided by the different agencies, comparing against: » Original projected outcomes » Physical needs » Psychosocial needs » Financial needs » Client and family satisfaction

- The nurse provides a link between all facets of the health care experience. This means coordinating care among the providers, nursing staff, physical and occupational therapists, rehabilitation facilities, home health care, and community resources.

- The case manager must be proactive for the client, balancing the impact of the illness against the cost of care. Increased knowledge of disease processes promotes early intervention and facilitates transition from acute to community-based care.

- Use of appropriate community agencies also will contain costs, because the monitoring of clients leads to better disease management.

TECHNOLOGY AND COMMUNITY NURSING

Overview

- Technological advances have led to drastic changes in the delivery of health care. The availability of new technologies results in a disruption of old delivery methods, while simultaneously creating new opportunities.
- The expense of new technology should be considered as implemented in the care of patients. Technology has had an impact on increasing life expectancy, yet also may lead to instances of ethical dilemmas in some situations.
- Nurses must remain appraised of new technologies in order to deliver optimal care. The introduction of new technologies can have a significant impact on communities, thus impacting health outcomes.

Informatics and Telehealth

- Informatics is the combination of nursing science with information and communication technologies in the delivery of nursing care.
  - Electronic records, databases, and billing are commonly used within current the health care industry. Hand-held computers and smartphones, geographic information systems, and the Internet all play a role in the delivery of health care.
  - Meetings can be held electronically. Chat rooms and asynchronous discussions can be used as an alternative delivery method for health education, to facilitate support groups, as a mechanism of peer collaboration, or in staff or student orientations/training.
- Telehealth is the delivery of quality health care through the use of technology.
  - Telehealth is particularly useful in rural areas. The ability to deliver specialized, skilled nursing through communications systems that transfers information easily between providers improves access to health care.
  - Home care services are increasingly using telehealth technologies in the delivery of client care. Emerging technology allows nurses to provide care to clients at home, while working from a central location, such as an office or health care agency. With the use of telehealth, however, it is important to balance the use of these services with actual hands-on care. A combination of these services is needed for optimal client outcomes.
  - Agencies transmitting or storing electronic health data must take measures to ensure confidentiality and security of client information.
  - Telecommunication technologies can transmit physical, audio, and visual data.
    - Transmission of physical data includes the following:
      - Blood pressure
      - Weight
      - Blood oxygenation
      - Blood glucose
      - Heart rate
      - Temperature
      - ECG results

- Transmission of audio data includes the following:
  - Voice conversation
  - Heart sounds
  - Lung sounds
  - Bowel sounds
- Transmission of visual data includes the following:
  - Images of wounds
  - Images of surgical incisions

PARTNERSHIPS WITH LEGISLATIVE BODIES

Overview

- Decisions and actions made by legislative bodies can have profound impacts on health. Health policy specifically addresses health issues within public policy.
- To facilitate needed change, it is important for nurses to stay informed of current policy and laws that influence both the health of the community and nursing practice. Nurses also should advocate for policies that protect public health or offer solutions to community problems.

Nursing's Role in Health Policy

- Change Agents – Advocate for needed change at the local, state, or federal level.
- Lobbyists – Persuade or influence legislators. Lobbying may be implemented by an individual, or collectively through professional nursing associations.
- Coalitions – Facilitation of goal achievement through the collaboration of two or more groups.
- Public Office – Serving society and advocating for change by influencing policy development through public service.

APPLICATION EXERCISES

1. A nurse is creating partnerships to address health needs within the community. The nurse should be aware that which of the following characteristics must exist for partnerships to be successful? (Select all that apply.)

_____ A. A leading partner with decision-making authority

_____ B. Flexibility among partners when considering new ideas

_____ C. Adherence of partners to ethical principles

_____ D. Varying goals for the different partners

_____ E. Willingness of partners to negotiate roles

2. A nurse is reviewing the various roles of a community health nurse. Which of the following is an example of a nurse functioning as a consultant?

A. Advocating for federal funding of local health screening programs

B. Updating state officials about health needs of the local community

C. Facilitating discussion of a client's ongoing needs with an interprofessional team

D. Performing health screenings for high blood pressure at a local health fair

3. A case management nurse at an acute care facility is conducting an initial visit with a client to identify needs prior to discharge home. After developing a working relationship with the client, the nurse is engaging in the referral process. Which of the following should be the first action by the nurse?

A. Monitor the client's satisfaction with the referral.

B. Provide client information to referral agencies.

C. Review available resources with the client.

D. Identify referrals that the client needs.

4. A nurse developing a community health program is determining barriers to community resource referrals. Which of the following is an example of a resource barrier?

A. Costs associated with services

B. Decreased motivation

C. Inadequate knowledge of resources

D. Lack of transportation

5. A nurse is working with a client who has systemic lupus erythematosus and recently lost her health insurance. Which of the following is an appropriate action by the nurse in the implementation phase of the case management process?

    A. Coordinating services to meet the client's needs

    B. Comparing outcomes with original goals

    C. Determining the client's financial constraints

    D. Clarifying roles of interprofessional team members

6. A nurse manager of a home health agency is preparing an in-service about informatics for a group of newly hired nurses. What should be included in this presentation? Using the ATI Active Learning Template: Basic Concept, complete this item to include the following:

    A. Related Content:
- Define informatics
- Define telehealth

    B. Underlying Principles:
- Two types of transmissible physical data
- Two types of transmissible audio data
- Two types of transmissible visual data

    C. Nursing Interventions:
- Three methods of incorporating technology into health care delivery

APPLICATION EXERCISES KEY

1. A. INCORRECT: Shared power must exist for a partnership to be successful.

    B. **CORRECT:** Flexibility must exist for a partnership to be successful.

    C. **CORRECT:** Integrity must exist for a partnership to be successful.

    D. INCORRECT: Shared goals must exist for a partnership to be successful.

    E. **CORRECT:** Negotiation must exist for a partnership to be successful.

    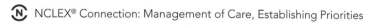 NCLEX® Connection: Management of Care, Concepts of Management

2. A. INCORRECT: This is an example of a nurse functioning as a change agent.

    B. **CORRECT:** This is an example of a nurse functioning as a consultant. Community health nurses serve as a consultant regarding the health care needs of individuals, families, and groups within the community served.

    C. INCORRECT: This is an example of a nurse functioning as a case manager.

    D. INCORRECT: This is an example of a nurse functioning as a caregiver.

    NCLEX® Connection: Management of Care, Collaboration with Interdisciplinary Team

3. A. INCORRECT: Monitoring the client's satisfaction with the referral is an appropriate action by the nurse. However, another action must occur first in the referral process.

    B. INCORRECT: Once the client agrees, providing client information to referral agencies is an appropriate action by the nurse. However, another action must occur first in the referral process.

    C. INCORRECT: Reviewing available resources with the client is an appropriate action by the nurse. However, another action must occur first in the referral process.

    D. **CORRECT:** Identifying referrals that the client needs is the first action the nurse should take in the referral process. Identifying the client's needs then allows the nurse and client to focus on specific needs while moving forward in the referral process.

    NCLEX® Connection: Management of Care, Establishing Priorities

4. A. **CORRECT:** Costs associated with services are an example of a resource barrier to community referrals.

    B. INCORRECT: Decreased motivation is an example of a client barrier to community referrals.

    C. INCORRECT: Inadequate knowledge of resources is an example of a client barrier to community referrals.

    D. INCORRECT: Lack of transportation is an example of a client barrier to community referrals.

    (N) NCLEX® Connection: Management of Care, Referrals

5. A. **CORRECT:** Coordinating services to meet the client's needs is an appropriate action by the nurse in the implementation phase of the case management process.

    B. INCORRECT: Comparing outcomes with original goals is an appropriate action by the nurse in the evaluation phase of the case management process.

    C. INCORRECT: Determining the client's financial constraints is an appropriate action by the nurse in the assessment phase of the case management process.

    D. INCORRECT: Clarifying roles of interprofessional team members is an appropriate action by the nurse in the planning phase of the case management process.

    (N) NCLEX® Connection: Management of Care, Case Management

6. *Using the ATI Active Learning Template: Basic Concept*

    A. Related Content
    - Informatics – the combination of nursing science with information and communication technologies in the delivery of nursing care
    - Telehealth – the delivery of quality health care through the use of technology

    B. Underlying Principles
    - Physical Data:
      - Blood pressure
      - Weight
      - Blood oxygenation
      - Blood glucose
      - Heart rate
      - Temperature
      - ECG results
    - Audio Data:
      - Voice conversation
      - Heart sounds
      - Lung sounds
      - Bowel sounds
    - Visual Data:
      - Wound images
      - Surgical incision images

    C. Nursing Interventions: Technology and health care delivery
    - Electronic records, databases, and billing
    - Internet availability of health information and education
    - Electronic meetings and chat rooms
    - Asynchronous discussions
    - Web-based support groups
    - Electronic orientation/training
    - Health care access in rural areas

    (N) NCLEX® Connection: Management of Care, Information Technology

Marquis, B. L., & Huston, C. J. (2012). *Leadership roles and management functions in nursing: Theory and application.* (7th ed.). Philadelphia: Lippincott Williams & Wilkins.

Nies, M., & McEwen, M. (2011). *Community/public health nursing: Promoting the health of populations* (5th ed.). St. Louis, MO: Saunders.

Stanhope, M., & Lancaster, J. (2010). *Foundations of nursing in the community* (3rd ed.). St. Louis, MO: Mosby.

Townsend, M. C. (2011). *Essentials of psychiatric mental health nursing: Concepts of care in evidence-based practice* (5th ed.). Philadelphia: F. A. Davis.

Varcarolis, E. M., Carson, V. B., & Shoemaker, N. C. (2010). *Foundations of psychiatric mental health nursing: A clinical approach* (6th ed.). St. Louis, MO: Saunders.

CONTENT_____ REVIEW MODULE CHAPTER _____

TOPIC DESCRIPTOR_____

Related Content (e.g. delegation, levels of prevention, advance directives)	Underlying Principles	Nursing Interventions
		› Who?
		› When?
		› Why?
		› How?

Appendix

CONTENT_____ REVIEW MODULE CHAPTER _____

TOPIC DESCRIPTOR_____

DESCRIPTION OF PROCEDURE:

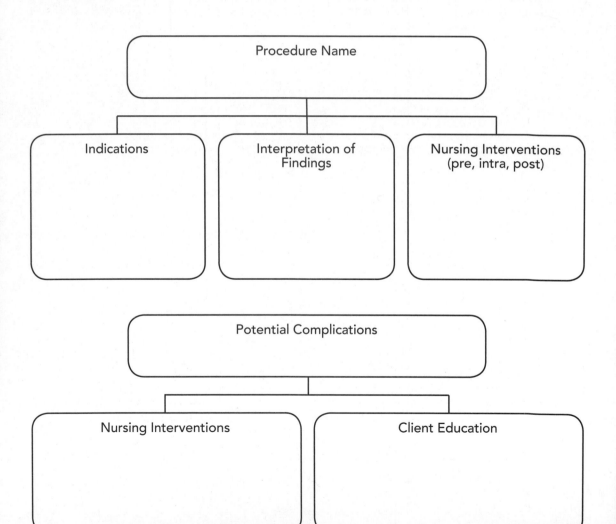

Appendix

CONTENT _____ REVIEW MODULE CHAPTER _____

TOPIC DESCRIPTOR_____

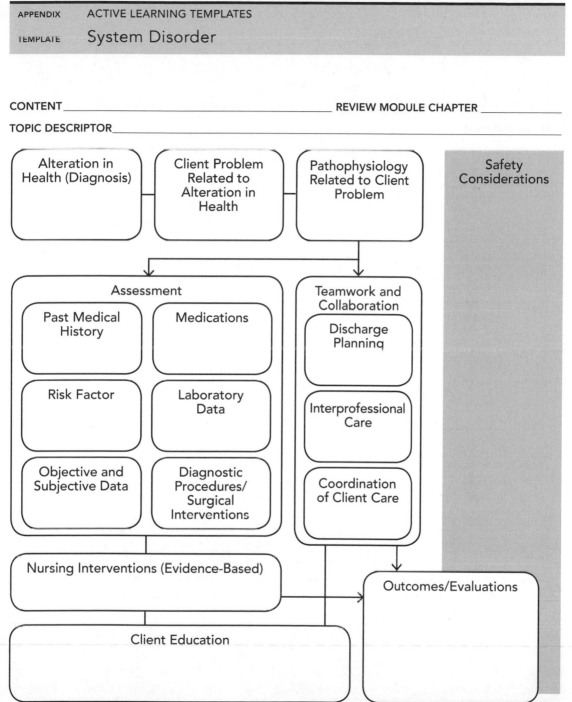

Appendix

CONTENT _____ REVIEW MODULE CHAPTER _____

TOPIC DESCRIPTOR _____

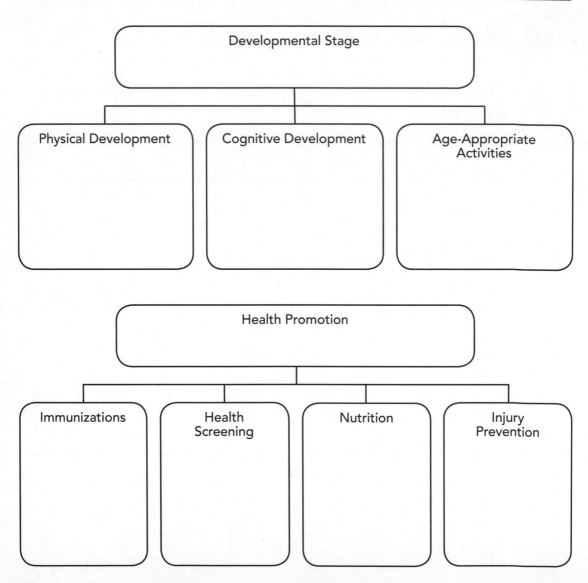

Developmental Stage

Physical Development

Cognitive Development

Age-Appropriate Activities

Health Promotion

Immunizations

Health Screening

Nutrition

Injury Prevention

APPENDIX ACTIVE LEARNING TEMPLATES

TEMPLATE Medication

CONTENT _____ REVIEW MODULE CHAPTER _____

TOPIC DESCRIPTOR_____

MEDICATION _____

EXPECTED PHARMACOLOGICAL ACTION:

Therapeutic Uses

Adverse Effects

Nursing Interventions

Contraindications

Client Education

Medication/Food Interactions

Medication Administration

Evaluation of Medication Effectiveness

Appendix

APPENDIX   ACTIVE LEARNING TEMPLATES

TEMPLATE   Nursing Skill

CONTENT _____ REVIEW MODULE CHAPTER _____

TOPIC DESCRIPTOR _____

DESCRIPTION OF SKILL:

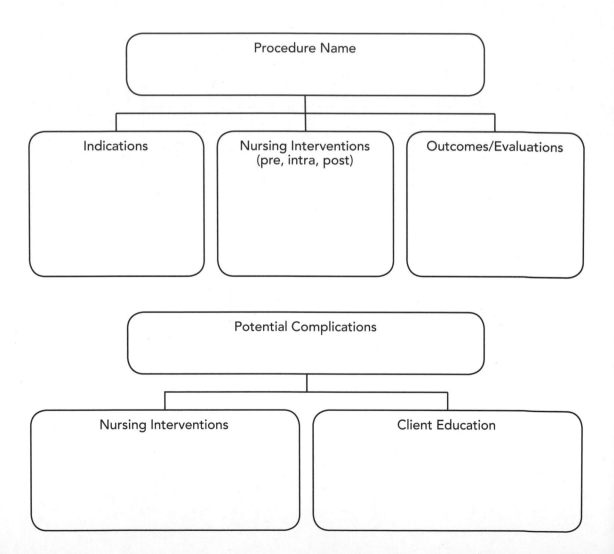

Appendix

CONTENT _____ REVIEW MODULE CHAPTER _____

TOPIC DESCRIPTOR _____

DESCRIPTION OF PROCEDURE:

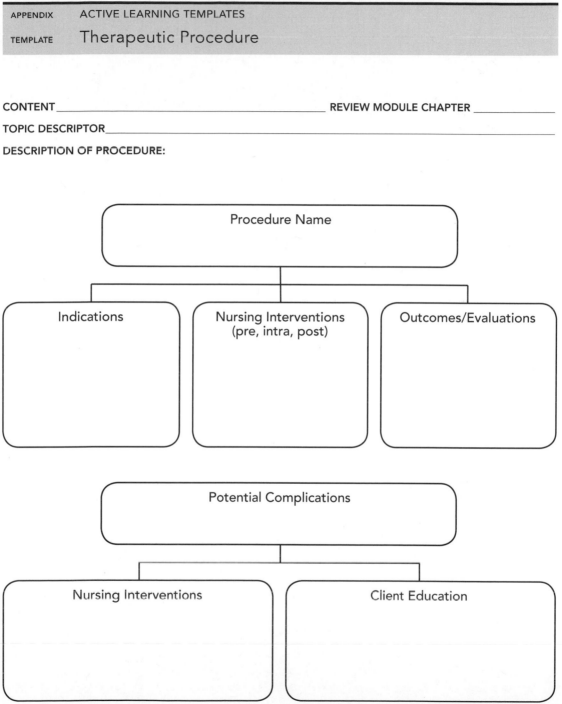

Procedure Name

Indications

Nursing Interventions
(pre, intra, post)

Outcomes/Evaluations

Potential Complications

Nursing Interventions

Client Education